FAT GONE

How 200 Pounds Vanished

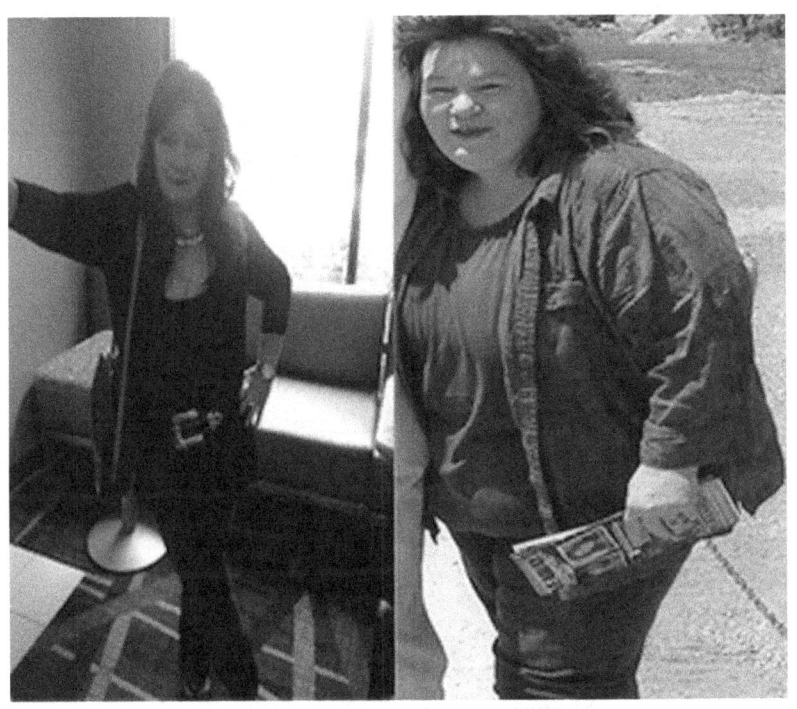

Cristie Will

Cristie Will

FAT GONE
How 200 Pounds Vanished
Copyright © 2015 by Cristie Will

FAT GONE
How 200 Pounds Vanished

Dedication

I want to dedicate this to my Late Husband Richard A. Will and my Mother Deanna Walton Dyer. I love and miss you both!
Also, I want to dedicate this book to everyone that struggles with their weight. God Bless you!

Acknowledgements

First off I want to thank my Creator, God my Lord and Savior. Without my Creator I would not have had the opportunity to have written this book.

I want to thank Mel for her continued support with ideas, with my book, health coaching and everyday life. Mel was with me through my darkest days and there were many of them.

I want to thank my daughter Lauren for being there when I needed her the most. Lauren was available at all hours day and night 24/7 if I needed her and that in itself is a huge comfort.

Forward

Cristie's been such an amazing example to me not only through her amazing spirit, but also through her incredible success. Before Cristie began focusing on her own health and weight loss, she had an intense belief that clean eating and living a nutritious lifestyle would heal, or at least relieve the effects of her husband Rich's cancer and the intense side effects. She strongly believed that had he followed a healthy eating regimen and lifestyle, he would not have had to go through the struggles that he endured. Unfortunately he didn't listen to her but listened to his doctors who prescribed highly toxic treatments.

After his death, she began to live the lifestyle she had come to so strongly believe in. I watched her transform her lifestyle and eating habits to such an extreme that she was able to get off all medications, lose 200 pounds and obtain a vibrancy that I haven't ever seen in my life. She has been such an amazing force and mentor in my life to become healthy and change my life. She has encouraged me and instructed me on how to go through a very healthy fasting regimen, change my eating habits, develop healthy sleep patterns, and focus on a positive life in general.

Cristie is someone who I regularly reach out to when I need encouragement, reminders, instruction and overall support when it comes to my healthy lifestyle, eating habits and emotional support. Cristie is a great mentor, teacher, role model and example for anyone who wants to live a life of health and well-being.

Maryellen Madden

Forward

How do I begin to express what a wonderful asset Cristie has been in my life. Observing her own life struggles with health and being able to overcome it has been rather inspiring! Through her trial and errors, along with the thorough amount of research in learning how to live the healthiest life, she has helped myself and others reach their healthiest potential. I can't thank her enough for teaching me how to eat properly and feel good, and to stop relying on medication for my ADD.

I truly believe anyone that taps into her resources will see what a gem she is to the health industry. She is a diamond in the rough because she understands the meaning of wellness and what it takes to attain that. If there's one person I trust with my health that would be Cristie. I really like that she focused on my specific health needs and understands that there's no one diet fits all plan. Not only does she help direct you into choosing a lifestyle that best suits you but she is that cheerleader you need when you feel it's just too tough. Yes it may feel like a struggle at first and yes with any new eating plans it can be overwhelming but trust me when you follow what she recommends she does know what she's talking about and you will never feel better if you follow her advice.

Thanks for your wisdom and encouragement, you have truly enriched my life.

Christopher Schneider

Introduction

This book is the result of finally succeeding in a true way to regain my health and lose 200 pounds at the age of 56. I not only lost the weight, but I restored my health from life threatening diseases, freeing myself of all medications and quit smoking.

I have been overweight most of my life and I have been the typical yoyo dieter. After all the struggles, tears and poor health I realized there is no magic pill to fix obesity or to regain vibrant health. I have been on or tried just about every diet, diet program, so called magic diet pills and powders on the market. In my experience most do not work and the ones that do are only a temporary fix.

I had lost hope year after year not to mention the thousands of dollars I have spent searching for the answer to my obesity issues but failed to find the solution once again. I was tired of the billions of dollars the weight loss industry is making playing on our emotions. I know I sure didn't mind spending the money for a solution fore I was at my wits end year after year fighting the weight loss battle.

I was so unhealthy with so many serious health issues that I had to lose weight. Every day things got a little better. Once I realized I just couldn't do it alone anymore is when I turned my life over to God, my creator.

We all have a certain threshold of pain and once we reach that threshold that is usually when change comes. I know once I hit my threshold of pain I couldn't take another second of misery and told myself I am done there is a better life waiting for me! Indeed I found a better life through good health and a whole lot less weight.

You can lose the weight even during menopause and you can quit smoking too. I always said I couldn't lose weight because I was going through menopause and I didn't want to quit smoking in fear of gaining even more weight, but I did quit smoking while going through menopause and I lost the weight.

I am hoping my book will help and inspire everyone that is struggling with their weight and looking for a healthy way to finally lose weight and keep it off.

I want to be the Health Coach that makes such a difference in people's lives that it becomes an domino effect. My hope is I help others and they in return reach out to help someone to help put an end to obesity.

You have what it takes to do this. I hope you will read this whole book and implement a plan to connect your dots to a happy healthy life.

Cristie Will

1
My Story
Growing up

I was born and raised in Hobbs, New Mexico, the middle daughter of five with four brothers. It was not easy with all those boys, but I wouldn't trade them for the world now that my brothers and I are grown. Growing up I would have gladly let you have any or all of my brothers for free.

I grew up in a pretty normal family back in the 1960's. There wasn't much in my small town for girls to do. They didn't have sports back then like they do now. All of my brothers played baseball and football.

Hobbs was a small transient town. The industry was and still is the oil patch. When things were good we would see an influx of people moving in and when things went south in the oil patch then the people would move on. The oil companies managed to transfer people in and out it felt like a lot. I would just become good friends with someone and their dad would get transferred. Because of this it seemed I was always lonely for a friend even though I had all those brothers.

I was an average sized kid as far as weight until I hit the fourth grade. I was 9 years old in the fourth grade and started my menstrual cycle. I had no idea what was wrong and too afraid to tell my mother. I thought I had something wrong with me. This was the year before we were shown the film on the birds and the bees, the male and female parts. This was the year my weight shot up from 70 pounds to 121. From 9 years old until now I struggled with my weight. That was the year my weight struggles began.

I remember in the fourth grade weighing in front of some kids in my class room and one girl went running back to the class room to tell the other students what I weighed. I outweighed a lot of the girls by about 5 pounds and I guess that was a lot. I was made fun of until I was into tears and because of this incident I never would get weighed in front of anyone again. To this day I don't like weighing in front of people for fear of still feeling overweight even though I am not.

By the time I was in the sixth grade I weighed 156 pounds at 5'2". My weight just continued to increase from the 4th grade on, but my height stayed at 5'2". My mom took me to the diet doctor, (that's what we called them back in the day), to help me. The diet doctor would basically prescribe appetite control pills, vitamins and water pills along with a laxative. I would lose some and gain it back. I went to the diet doctor on and off for about 15 years getting the same results – lose the weight then gain it back time and time again.

I was ridiculed and bullied all my life because I was overweight. My parents took us to see the Grand Canyon in Arizona and my brothers said I made the canyon by falling down. This is just an example of things said. They were kidding, but it still was very painful.

After the fourth grade I got to where I quit riding my bicycle because kids would yell out at me "get off that bike your tires are flat fatso".

When I was in the sixth grade this male classmate that walked on his tiptoes would say "Every time you take a step the ground shakes". Thinking about it now I can laugh, but being 12 years old and wanting to fit in caused me to go into depression and eat more.

Almost every single day from the fourth grade until I graduated from High School someone would say "Fatty fatty two by four can't get through the bathroom door". The tears would well in my eyes and I would muster getting by the kids saying this. I honestly don't know how I made it with all the cruel words, but I did.

When I entered into the seventh grade we had to walk across the street for a math class in another building. Every day going to my math class a male classmate would call me Bear, he would say "You eat so much just like a Bear" and he would growl like a bear and just repeat this until I was in the classroom. Some of the other kids would laugh and chime in as well. I would cry every day and begged to go to a different school. Looking back even if I went to a different school it would not have been any different. This was bullying, but had not been labeled yet. Adults looked at it as kids being kids or at least that was my experience.

I was lucky enough to be accepted into a sorority and it wasn't because I was popular like the other girls, it was because I had popular good looking brothers. At the time I liked it because otherwise no way would I have a chance in hell getting accepted.

My sorority had a dance and I couldn't find a date. I asked my brothers friends just so I could have an escort and to have someone to get my picture taken with at the dance, but not even my brother's popularity helped that. Year after year our sorority dances I went alone and no pictures.

High School Prom nights were pretty much the same story as the sorority dances. I never could find a date to prom, so I didn't go to any of the prom dances. I look back now and wished I would have gone. I know there were others that didn't have dates and went anyways. I just felt so isolated and worthless during this time in my life.

I Graduated from high school and started going to the junior college, but soon dropped out because it wasn't much better as far as being able to go to class without hurtful remarks. By this time my self-esteem was rock bottom and I didn't feel worthy of anything and flunked out. Later in life little by little I did manage to get my college education.

First Marriage and Beyond

In 1982 I was baptized in the church and was looking to marry. I didn't date much and met my first husband at church and married him. I thought he would make a great husband and father, after all I wanted the white picket fence with the husband and kids.

I only dated my husband for two months and ran off and got married. I was 25 at the time and all my friends were married. My friends were all having kids, so I wanted kids. I was afraid I would never be able to have kids, so I married the first chance I got, to be sure to have kids.

I got married in 1983 and my weight was hovering around 180 lbs. A couple of years later I had my first child in 1985 and my weight spiraled out of control. After the birth of my first child I weighed 250. In 1989 I had my second child and ballooned up to 305 lbs. I would go on diet after diet and lose 30 to 50 pounds and gain it all back again and again.

My middle name should have been diet because at any given day I was on a diet. Every time a new diet pill would come out. I was always one of the first to buy it and try it only to be let down and just heartbroken once again.

I was miserable in my marriage and would have gotten divorced, but the church didn't believe in divorce and I didn't want to disgrace my family further. Even though I was so miserable in my marriage I do not regret it because I have two beautiful children.

In October 1990 I got a phone call from my baby sitter telling me that my daughter told her my husband was molesting my daughter. I was in utter shock that this good Christian man could do such a thing, those were my thoughts. I realize now that good and bad people come in all walks of life. At first he denied his actions, but at the end of the day he admitted it and we got a divorce. I couldn't understand this and went into a deep depression. I felt hopeless and helpless. My house with the white picket fence was gone. My weight continued to rise up to 330.

After my divorce I stayed single and worked for the family construction business until my parents sold this business in March 1996. This business was my grandfathers and had been in the family for 60 years. Selling the business was like a death in the family. For the next year I was depressed and never left the house except to take kids to and from school, the grocery store and to do necessary errands.

I finally got sick and tired of the pain I was in, physically and especially emotionally, so I started walking and cutting back on my eating. I was starting to lose weight. I had to find a job and wanted a change, so I moved to Loveland, Colorado. My youngest brother was living in Fort Collins, Colorado going to Colorado State University and wanted me to come check the area out to start over. With nothing to lose and everything to gain I moved to Colorado.

I went to work for a small construction company as their receptionist in Loveland. A year later they promoted me to their bookkeeper. I worked for this construction company for the next 12 years.

I continued to walk and eat healthy and lose weight. I lost 180 pounds and was ready to date after being single for 10 years.

Not really knowing anyone to date I decided to sign up for online dating in 2001. Online dating was relatively new or at least it was to me. This online dating was a real experience and was difficult at the time for me because of the rejection I had encountered in the past. Still having self-esteem issues the rejection was hard to stomach. Since I didn't date in high school I didn't know how to date or what to expect.

I met and dated 18 different men online. All of them but 2 were only one or two dates. Number 18 was the love of my life, Rich was his name. I remember not wanting to go out with Rich, because I thought he was too old for me. I met Rich out for dinner and we closed the place down that night. We just hit it off and talked and talked about everything. We dated 2 ½ years and then married.

I finally got to experience what most people in high school experience and that is simply really living and experiencing what life is about such as dating, traveling, attending concerts and being able to bend over and tie my shoes. This is due to my finally losing so much weight and giving me a temporary lift with my self-esteem.

I thought my pain in life ended and it was all good since I lost my weight. I thought at the time only really fat people like me lived in hell on earth. I was so miserable I couldn't see anything, but my pain. The emotional baggage and pain I had experienced had blinded me so much that I could not see that all people have setbacks and problems. I finally learned setbacks and problems aren't because of obesity only. Unfortunately it took me many years to figure this out.

Second Marriage

Rich and I traveled quite a bit in the first few years of our marriage and I had the time of my life. We ate and drank at all these different places and before long I allowed myself to gain the weight back. My husband was so good to me and very supportive. I would repeatedly lose 30 pounds and gain that back on and off. 30 pounds is a drop in the bucket at my weight.

In 2007 my husband Rich had throat cancer surgery and got through that ok. I quit smoking in 2008 and didn't gain any weight which was a miracle in itself. I quit smoking because I needed to and with Rich having throat cancer I thought I would quit in hopes of him quitting smoking too, but he had not.

In 2009 I started going through menopause. Dealing with the hot flashes along with all the excess weight was almost enough to send me down the river. My husband was a trooper even though I about froze him out of the bedroom. I had the ceiling fan going and a floor fan going and Rich never complained.

In 2010 we were in Jackson Hole, WY on our anniversary and Rich woke up on 10-10-10 sounding like he had laryngitis. We came home after a four day trip and Rich still had his laryngitis. Rich was in sales and needed his voice. Rich had a 3 week trip coming up that he needed to go to, so I told him to go to the doctor and see if maybe they have something for laryngitis. On October 14, 2010 Rich goes to the doctor for his checkup. It was his birthday.

Friday October 15, 2010 the doctor called and said he wanted Rich to go see a specialist on Monday that he had a blockage and didn't know what it was. Monday October 18, 2010 comes and we go to this doctor and the doctor said "Rich you have lung cancer". Talk about getting the breath knocked out of you that is what it felt like. Taken by total surprise. I asked my husband if he had been feeling bad or anything unusual and he said no.

November 1, 2010 was when Rich started his first Chemotherapy treatment and he breezed right through the first rounds on the same Chemotherapy. After his first round of Chemotherapy he goes in to have scans and shows the cancer has shrunk.

Rich now starts another round of Chemotherapy treatment, but it's starting to affect him with loss of appetite and a bit of fatigue. He goes in for more scans and his cancer has shrunk some more, but not gone.

Rich now starts Radiation while starting another round of Chemotherapy. The radiation is really taking a toll on him. The radiation was so bad that it burnt his throat and chest area to the point of not being able to swallow. I lost it in the doctor's office saying "This is killing my husband he is not a number! He can't keep doing this aggressive radiation along with Chemotherapy, change something now!!!!" They cut back for a couple of weeks on his radiation.

Rich resumes and completes his radiation along with three bouts of chemotherapy. It's been 13 months of pretty much straight treatment and we go in for scans with the radiologist. We finally got great news the cancer was gone.

After finding out that Rich had lung cancer, I packed on more weight for the next 16 months. First I started eating more because I am an emotional eater and I would turn to food out of fear of what was probably going to happen to my husband.

Rich would come by my office to take me to lunch from time to time and if I had eaten then he would not eat and I never knew when he might want to go to lunch, so even if I had already had lunch I would tell him I hadn't and go eat again with him so he would eat. This is the only time I don't regret gaining the weight.

October 14, 2011 Rich was on a trip in California and this was his birthday. I had to call him to tell him that his mother passed on his birthday. This just tore my heart out for Rich. Rich had already been through heck and back and then to lose his mom while he was out of town on his birthday was too much to bear.

Rich was a real trooper and never one time complained about what he was going through.

Cristie Will

January 14, 2012 Rich had gone to the hospital and we found out his cancer had spread to other organs in his body and about 5 weeks later he passed, February 20, 2012.

Needless to say I was lost in a fog after losing my husband. We had Rich's funeral about 5 days later and I couldn't have done it without the help of his kids and family. Rich's sons and daughter in laws don't get any better. They all stepped up to the plate without asking and got things done right. They all were an absolute Godsend for me along with my family and best friend, Maryellen.

By this time my weight was around 331 and I felt horrible not to mention I looked worse than I felt. It would take me an hour every morning just to get out of bed and be able to walk without pain. After Rich's death I didn't want to get out of bed not only because of the ongoing physical pain, but now I had the emotional pain of loss of my husband that was so vibrant and way too young to die.

April 11, 2012 I get a letter from Rich's ex-wife's attorney suing me to continue paying her alimony plus other things. I was in shock I was still grieving the loss of my husband. The lawsuit finally ended. For three years it was one thing after another that was difficult and painful. Somehow I made it through the worst period of my life and honestly I didn't think this hell would ever end, but it did.

Life is full of ups and downs. I learned I am more resilient than I ever thought possible and that by hanging through the tough times life would get better. Now life is much better than I ever could have dreamed!

The Emotional and Physical Pain of Being Obese

Along with the obvious health challenges, being obese has other harsh realities. I would get stared at everywhere I went and I could almost read their minds. When I would go to a restaurant I could feel people just watching every bite of food I ate and watch me take every step out the door waddling. I am sure they thought how disgusting I was, so fat stuffing more food down my throat into my swollen body.

I felt like I should have been in a carnival as the freak show of the day. I was so self-conscious knowing the way I looked and felt. I wanted to slip in and out without being noticed, so I always wore dark colors like black or dark navy. What I didn't realize I was so fat I couldn't slip in or out unnoticed anywhere at any time.

It was a chore to tie my shoes, put socks on or to even bend down. It was like finding gold once I got my panty hose on, if I could find them large enough. These are everyday easy things for most people unless you are obese or have a different disability.

Getting in and out of cars is hard and some cars I couldn't fit in. It's surprising I didn't have a wreck driving. I was so fat that I had to push the seat so far back that I had to strain to reach the gas and brake pedals.

Oh and flying was probably the hardest. I was so fat I couldn't get the seat buckled and I was not about to draw attention to myself and ask for an extension. I realize now that was wrong and put others and myself in more danger by not asking and wished I had taken a deep breath and asked for an extension to my seat belt.

I could get in the bath tub, but had to have assistance to get out. It was way too painful and embarrassing to ask my husband to help me out.

Bathing was darn near impossible, so I only showered and it was difficult. It was so hard reaching my private areas that I asked my husband for one of those removable shower heads so I could just point the water where it needed to go. I didn't tell my husband that I wanted it because I was so fat, but I bet he knew that is why I asked for a new shower head.

I guess the regular scales only went up to about 300 at the hospital because they took me back to the flat bed scale to weigh me. Then when the nurses would take my blood pressure they would have to find the largest cuff to fit around my arm. Drawing blood on me was another issue. My arms were so fat I had to have the needle in my hand, which was the only place they could find a vein.

In 1989 I had to have a C-Section for the birth of my son. I was huge and I felt like a big fat whale laying out in the open on a table in the operating room. I was completely naked and people going in and out of the room staring at me. My body was so big I could not see the doctor standing at the end of the bed because my belly was in the way.

In 2010 I had to have my appendix removed, and I woke up crying uncontrollably because I was still alive. All I could think about was how fat I was and that everyone in the surgery room probably came over to look at such a disgusting fat woman. I didn't want to look at anyone.

All the photo shopped pictures we see on magazines and television sends us all into hopelessness because no one has that perfect of a body or complexion. This just adds another layer to the emotional toll for most, but especially the obese. Seeing these images causes that vicious cycle of trying to lose only to fail once again. Now we start telling ourselves what fat losers we are. What we say and tell ourselves we seem to become, so the cycle just continues over and over as the weight on our bodies climbs to an all-time high.

What many people don't realize is that being obese is a disability and that it's not as easy as just quit eating so much. If it were that easy we would all be slim and the billions made on weight loss would be a thing of the past.

Obesity is a disease that causes other diseases like high blood pressure and diabetes, and it is no laughing matter. It's time we all take a stand to put an end to this epidemic that is causing untimely deaths at a younger and younger age.

I cried myself to sleep many nights in so much physical and emotional pain. It seemed no matter what I tried it just didn't work. I was so unhealthy and in tremendous pain I prayed to God to take me.

Until a person has lived being obese they will never know the true pain of being obese.

Cristie Will

Pictures of me at various functions and times in my life. As you can see I was obese in all of these photos. I have many more. I did my best to not be in pictures.

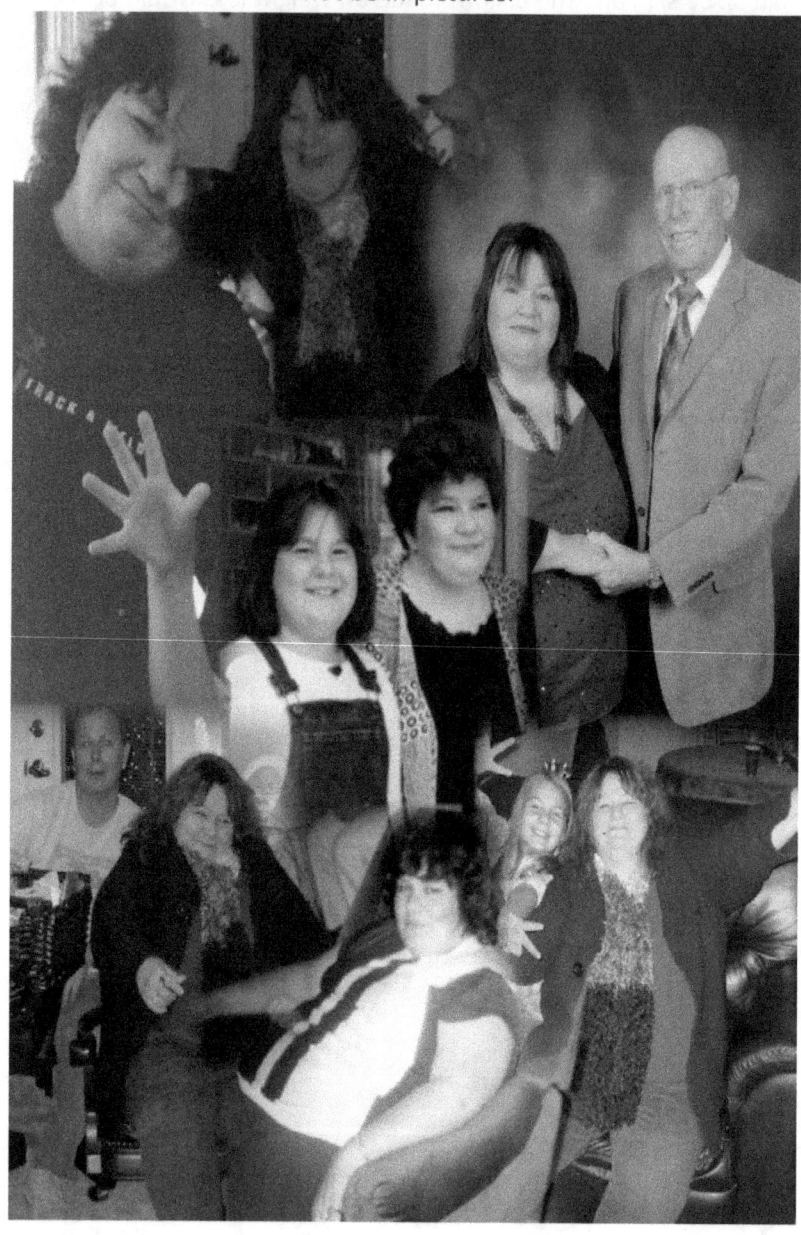

Pictures of me at various functions and times in my life. As you can see I am a lot thinner and happier in all of these photos. I have many more. I don't mind being in pictures now.

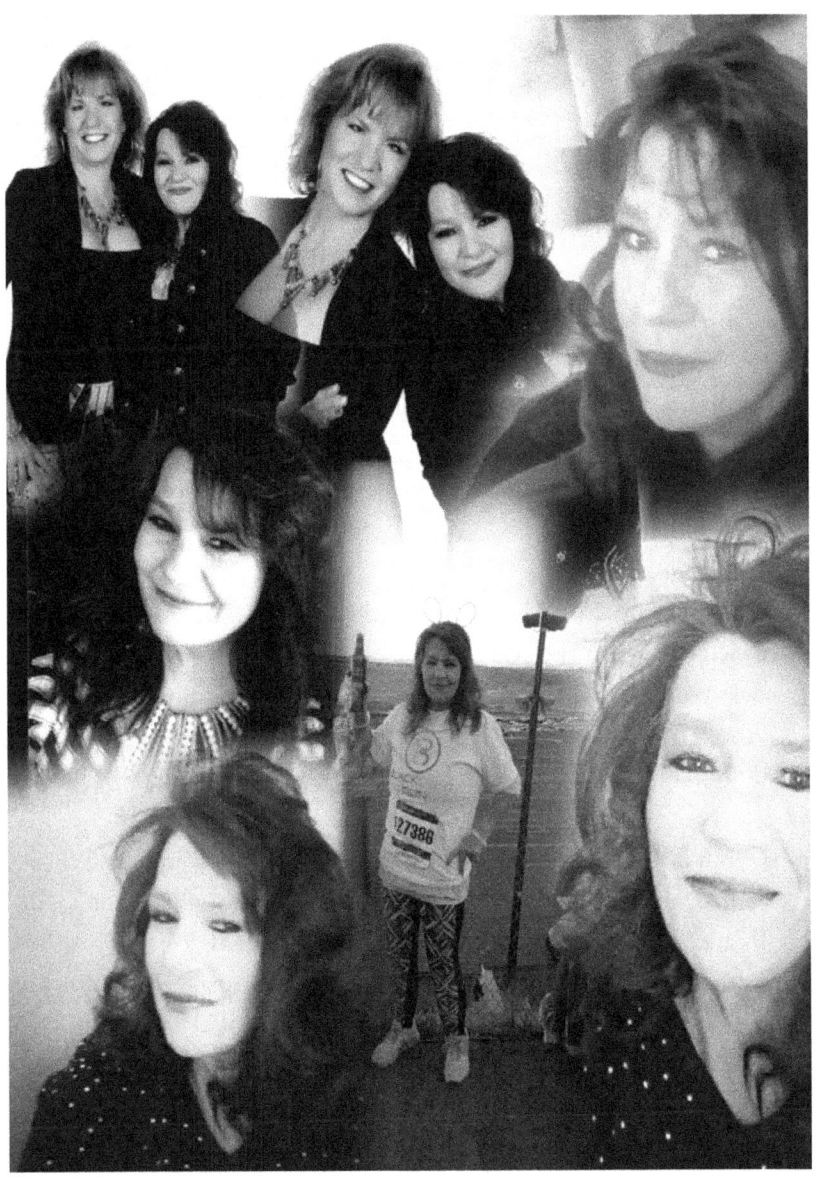

2
Smoking and Menopause

Smoking

My friend that lived across the street from me growing up would take her mom's cigarettes and we would smoke them. This was my first experience with smoking at the age of nine. Then it graduated to me taking my mom's cigarettes so we wouldn't get caught we thought. This way we traded off taking cigarettes from each other's moms, until one day my mom caught us.

My mother sent my friend home and told her mom. The next thing my mom did was make me smoke in front of her, my dad and my grandmother. I choked up and got sick plus really embarrassed, so I quit. I did not take another cigarette or puff of a cigarette until I was sixteen.

Sixteen came around and my weight would balloon up and down in a vicious circle. The word on the street was that smoking would help you lose weight, so I signed right up for that one and smoked. I thought I was being so sneaky, but my mom knew. It seemed my mom knew everything and she did when it pertained to her kids.

I would smoke in my room with the window open and slide the ashtray under my bed thinking I wouldn't get caught, what a laugh that was. My mom told me one day just come on out here and smoke with us. I had the look of utter shock. I remember thinking how does she know I open my window. She said I can see the smoke flowing out under your door. I started smoking in front of my parents and very hard at first, but managed to do it. At this point I didn't care I wanted to lose weight and I had the tool, or so I thought.

I kept smoking until I got pregnant with my first child in 1985 and quit during pregnancy. After the birth of my daughter I soon began smoking again. I smoked until I got pregnant with my second child in 1988 and gave birth in 1989. Once again I resumed smoking after the birth of my son because now I really needed to lose weight.

I quit smoking a couple of times other than during my pregnancy for about a year at a time and would soon light up again. Looking back now I realized all the things going on in my life and all the things missing in my life caused me to turn to cigarettes again. Now food and cigarettes were my crutches.

Both my parents smoked, but none of my brothers smoked. This puts the squash on blaming ones parents since it seems not only myself and society blames everything on our parents. Yes our upbringing plays a role in our life, but we still make choices such as to smoke or not to smoke. I of course took up the smoking.

Smoking along with my huge body was literally choking off my air supply, or at least that was how I was feeling not long before I quit. Each puff I would take it was like I would lose my breath and my 330 pound body was suffocating.

I decided I had to do something or prepare for an early death. I started and failed miserably dieting every day of my life. Since I could not lose the weight I threw my cigarettes away and never picked up another going on 6 years now. I knew that by quitting I would probably gain more weight, but felt I had no choice.

Amazingly I did not gain any more weight, but it's probably because I was already so big that my small frame just couldn't take another pound. My goal was to quit for a year so that I could get use to not smoking and deal with the issues of not smoking then figure a way to lose some weight for my health reasons.

The year rolls around and it's 2010 and still obese thinking I need to take my weight issues seriously now and lose. I gave every excuse in the book as to when I would start to lose weight. I decided ok I will go on my wedding anniversary October 11, 2010 and when I get back I am going to do it that's it

As I mentioned in my story October 2010 is when my husband was diagnosed with lung cancer and I turned to my biggest crutch, food. I of course started the weight gain switch until I reached weighing 330. I look back now and thankful I didn't take up smoking again not only for my health, but for my husband's health too.

We can do anything we put our minds to do. I know with myself when I accomplish things that are next to impossible is when I have had enough by reaching my threshold of pain. I know I have to get to the point the pain is so severe in my life that I say enough is enough.

Once I reach the enough is enough stage then it's so easy to do what I set out and it's all because the pain of going back is too great. This final time I decided to quit smoking there was no question. I didn't even need to buy hard candy or anything I was just done.

When I quit smoking it was like I never smoked in my life. I never missed or even thought about cigarettes except every once in a while I would think about how long I had not had a cigarette.

Since we are all bio individuals when you quit smoking it will be different than what and how I quit smoking as well. This is what it will take in a nut shell.

Quitting Smoking

When you are ready to quit smoking go through the reasons why you need and want to quit smoking. Make the decision to quit smoking and don't look back. Don't worry about gaining weight, if you do just know that is your next obstacle to tackle. Ask yourself what it is going to take to quit smoking once and for all. Your health will improve, you will save money, your skin will improve and not age as fast, your family won't be around your second hand smoke just to name a few of the benefits.

Here are statistics to help you realize why you need to be serious about smoking. My hope is for you to quit smoking without medications, but if that is what it takes then you should do what is necessary for you to quit smoking.

Smoking

Cigarette smoking is the number one cause of preventable disease and death worldwide. Smoking-related diseases claim over 393,000 American lives each year. Smoking cost the United States over $193 billion in 2004, including $97 billion in lost productivity and $96 billion in direct health care expenditures, or an average of $4,260 per adult smoker.[1]

Key Facts about Smoking

- Cigarette smoke contains over 7,000 chemicals, 69 of which are known to cause cancer.[19] Smoking is directly responsible for approximately 90 percent of lung cancer deaths and approximately 80-90 percent of COPD (emphysema and chronic bronchitis) deaths.[2]
- Among adults who have ever smoked, 70% started smoking regularly at age 18 or younger, and 86% at age 21 or younger.[3]
- Among current smokers, chronic lung disease accounts for 73 percent of smoking-related conditions. Even among smokers who have quit chronic lung disease accounts for 50 percent of smoking-related conditions.[4]
- Smoking harms nearly every organ in the body, and is a main cause of lung cancer and chronic obstructive pulmonary disease (COPD, including chronic bronchitis and emphysema). It is also a cause of coronary heart disease, stroke and a host of other cancers and diseases.[5]

Smoking Rates among Adults & Youth

- In 2009, an estimated 46.6 million, or 20.6 percent of adults (aged 18+) were current smokers.[6]
- Men tend to smoke more than women. In 2009, 23.5 percent of men currently smoked compared to 17.9 percent of females.[7]
- Prevalence of current smoking in 2009 was highest among non-Hispanic whites (22.2%) intermediate among non-Hispanic blacks (21.3%), and lowest among Hispanics (14.5%) and Asians (12.0%).[8]
- In 2009, 19.5 percent of high school students were current smokers.[9] Over 5 percent of middle school students were current smokers in 2009.[10]

- **Smoking during Pregnancy**

- Smoking in pregnancy accounts for an estimated 20 to 30 percent of low-birth weight babies, up to 14 percent of preterm deliveries, and some 10 percent of all infant deaths. Even apparently healthy, full-term babies of smokers have been found to be born with narrowed airways and reduced lung function.[11]
- In 2005, 10.7 percent of all women smoked during pregnancy, down almost 45 percent from 1990.[12]
- Neonatal health-care costs attributable to maternal smoking in the U.S. have been estimated at $366 million per year, or $704 per maternal smoker.[13]

- **Facts about Quitting Smoking**

- Nicotine is the ingredient in cigarettes that causes addiction. Smokers not only become physically addicted to nicotine; they also link smoking with many social activities, making smoking an extremely difficult addiction to break.[14]
- In 2009, an estimated 49.9 million adults were former smokers. Of the 46.6 million current adult smokers, 46.7 percent stopped smoking at least 1 day in the preceding year because they were trying to quit smoking completely.[15]
- Quitting smoking often requires multiple attempts. Using counseling or medication alone increases the chance of a quit attempt being successful; the combination of both is even more effective.[16]
- There are seven medications approved by the U.S. Food and Drug Administration to aid in quitting smoking. Nicotine patches, nicotine gum and nicotine lozenges are available over-the-counter, and a nicotine nasal spray and inhaler are currently available by prescription. Buproprion SR (Zyban) and varenicline (Chantix) are non-nicotine pills.[17]

- Individual, group and telephone counseling are effective. Telephone quitline counseling is widely available and is effective for many different groups of smokers.18

- Information obtained from the American Lung Association. See Citations/Index/Resources for complete source listing.

Menopause

Here come's menopause just when I didn't need it most. I had quit smoking and battling my weight. It was already hard enough to lose weight and then topping it off with menopause was just like my system had turned off losing weight.

I always heard and read that it was darn near impossible to lose weight in menopause. The answer to this is yes and no to losing weight during menopause. I did and so can you.

Here comes the spotting, then sporadic periods, the mood swings intensify and then the hot flashes. Come on Mother Nature what's next was my question.

I guess it's not enough stress on our bodies to carry babies that stretch our bodies not to mention the change in our whole body chemistry. I must add though it was worth everything carrying that precious baby that God gives us.

The fans are blazing in the bedroom at night, the covers coming off and on all night, tossing and turning. It seems a good night's sleep was a thing in the past from the time I gave birth to my first child until menopause is done.

Needless to say I quit smoking about the time my menopause kicking in. There were times I thought I must be crazy.

When my paternal grandmother went through menopause she was all over the map with her emotions and actions. I remember asking my mother what is wrong with Mammie and my mom said oh she is crazy going through the change. When my maternal grandmother went through menopause she had no visible changes. No one ever knew when she went through the change. My paternal grandmother took medications for menopause and my maternal grandmother did not take anything. I don't think the medications had that big of a difference I think it boils down to the differences we all have because we are bio individuals.

Next the years of my mother's menopause. My mother had the most visible issues. I drove over to my parents' home. I get ready to get out of my car and my mother is banging the solid glass storm door against the brick trying to break the glass door. With no success my mother proceeds trying to break the glass door with a hammer.

After my mother trying to break the glass door with two attempts she realized she had a problem. Realizing this she went to the doctor. When my mother talks to her doctor about this issue, he said be thankful you realized you had the problem because most women don't realize they are having hormonal issues and blame others for their problems.

My mother started taking hormones and went through years of getting her hormones regulated with medications.

Here comes my time for menopause and I fear having issues like my paternal grandmother and mother. I hoped to go through menopause like my maternal grandmother, so I decided to not take hormones in hopes that maybe that was the difference.

During my menopause I found I didn't have near the mood swings my mother and grandmother had and I didn't put on the extra weight. What I did have was the hot flashes. I didn't have the night sweats though. I kept going through menopause without medications because I was told that if I took the medications I would never go through menopause and that if I got off the medications I would then go through menopause. Having learned that I chose no medications other than natural supplements.

Since I don't take any medications I supplement with natural hormone replacement therapy with supplements, eating healthy, exercise and meditation.

I am still going through menopause. My hot flashes have just about gone away since I started taking supplements and living healthier.

When I decided to lose my excess weight and get healthy I was right in the middle of menopause. You can lose the weight during menopause by taking the healthy approach, so I urge you not to let menopause keep you from your healthy weight loss and life.

We are all different and everything affects us differently, so I urge you to consult your physician before starting any kind of health changes.

Remember this too shall pass and hang in there. You can and will whip this too.

Information for Menopause

Symptoms

In the months or years leading up to menopause (perimenopause), you might experience these signs and symptoms:

- Irregular periods
- Vaginal dryness
- Hot flashes
- Night sweats
- Sleep problems
- Mood changes
- Weight gain and slowed metabolism
- Thinning hair and dry skin
- Loss of breast fullness

It's possible, but very unusual, to menstruate every month right up to your last period. More likely, you'll experience some irregularity in your periods.

Skipping periods during perimenopause is common and expected. Often, menstrual periods will occur every two to four months during perimenopause, especially one to two years before menopause. Despite irregular periods, pregnancy is possible. If you've skipped a period but aren't sure you've started the menopausal transition, you may want to determine whether you're pregnant.

When to see a doctor

Starting at perimenopause, schedule regular visits with your doctor for preventive health care and any medical concerns. Continue getting these appointments during and after menopause.

Preventive health care can include recommended screenings at menopause, such as a colonoscopy, mammography, lipid screening, thyroid testing (if suggested by your history), breast and pelvic exams. Always seek medical advice if you have bleeding from your vagina after

Cristie Will

menopause.

Information obtained from the Mayo Clinic. See
Citations/Index/Resources

Causes Menopause can result from:
- **Natural decline of reproductive hormones.** As you approach your late 30s, your ovaries start making less estrogen and progesterone — the hormones that regulate menstruation — and your fertility declines.

  In your 40s, your menstrual periods may become longer or shorter, heavier or lighter, and more or less frequent, until eventually — on average, by age 51 — your ovaries stop producing eggs, and you have no more periods.

- **Hysterectomy.** A hysterectomy that removes your uterus but not your ovaries (partial hysterectomy) usually doesn't cause immediate menopause. Although you no longer have periods, your ovaries still release eggs and produce estrogen and progesterone. But surgery that removes both your uterus and your ovaries (total hysterectomy and bilateral oophorectomy) does cause menopause, without any transitional phase. Your periods stop immediately, and you're likely to have hot flashes and other menopausal signs and symptoms, which can be severe, as these hormonal changes occur abruptly rather than over several years.

- **Chemotherapy and radiation therapy.** These cancer therapies can induce menopause, causing symptoms such as hot flashes during or shortly after the course of treatment. The halt to menstruation (and fertility) is not always permanent following chemotherapy, so birth control measures may still be desired.

- **Primary ovarian insufficiency.** About 1 percent of women experience menopause before age 40 (premature menopause). Menopause may result from primary ovarian insufficiency — when your ovaries fail to produce normal levels of reproductive hormones

— stemming from genetic factors or autoimmune disease. But often no cause can be found. For these women, hormone therapy is typically recommended at least until the natural age of menopause in order to protect the brain, heart and bones.

Information obtained from the Mayo Clinic. See
Citations/Index/Resources

3
Relationships

Communication for all

Our relationships are the most important part of our lives. Our relationships aren't just about our spouse, boyfriend, girlfriend or significant other. Relationships are with every walk of life such as parents, siblings, doctors, store clerks, our pets and our children just to name a few. Having said this about all relationships, the most important relationships are our spouse, family, boyfriend/girlfriend or significant other.

Having open communication within your relationships is so important because without that your life will be out of balance in one form or another.

We should not assume what the other person thinks. When we start assuming then the problems begin with hurt feelings, anger, frustration, disrespect and last but not least the resentment starts to build. Not necessarily in this order or these exact emotions.

Open communication starts with thinking about the other person with kindness and love. Treat them the way you want to be treated. Yes we will mess up from time to time, but it's not the end. Always think about what you are going to say before speaking to avoid misunderstandings and potential arguments turning into grudges.

Always be mindful that just one wrong negative word can destroy a relationship. Our tongues are the most powerful tool we have. With our tongues we can heal or we can destroy a person and or relationship. Our tongues can give us peace or unrest. Choose words wisely and make your life a loving peaceful one.

To have that clear communication make eye contact without distractions. The distractions displays disrespect and invariably you won't hear what was said and then the mistakes appear, because not hearing what was communicated.

You need to make time each week to listen and communicate without judgment. If you have judgment then the communication will be cut off. It's that simple pertaining to judgment.

When someone goes above and beyond doing things for you or giving you things be sure to acknowledge them and thank them. If you do not do this then the above and beyond doing and giving from them will drop off and even stop. You will be perceived as not caring and expecting it.

Always speak up about your feelings and any actions that make you feel uneasy in any way such as hurt, guilty or even stressed. Listen to your gut instincts if it doesn't feel right take appropriate action right then and there so you can avoid the blaming game that often turns to isolating yourself or the other person.

Do you understand the other person in your relationships needs? If you are unsure then get sure. Be open and share your preferences on everything like your strengths and weaknesses down to your pet peeves. This is the real way to avoid misunderstandings or at least most of them.

Do you know the desires, visions and goals of your important relationships? If you do not know their visions or goals make it a point to find out. By finding out is another solution to avoid more miscommunication.

Something as simple as bringing home flowers to your wife that she is allergic to. This action will speak volumes to her especially if she told you she was allergic to them. This will tell her you don't care enough to listen and you got her flowers because you felt you had to not because you wanted to. This in turn causes a huge chain reaction of hurt feelings, anger, resentment and blame. Too many of these things that you may think are small build and can turn into huge problems even divorce if it's with your spouse.

Do you rephrase what was being said? It's important to rephrase what's being said to be sure you understand one another to avoid extra problems. This always shows that you care and are truly listening to the other person's needs and desires.

Remember to smile. Smiling is communicating and can make anyone's day brighter. You never know that smile could save someone's life. Smiling can be more powerful because it's an action and actions are more powerful than words.

By creating healthy and long lasting relationships takes work. Communication is the key to your great relationships. This does not mean you will agree with everyone all the time. We are all different and we will like something's the same and something's will be totally different, but there is always a healthy compromise when necessary. Do not take advantage of the people you care about fore they may just not be there one day.

At the end of the day smile, give a helping hand when needed and speak kindly and your life will improve significantly on this alone. We all want to feel good and these actions will do just that. Also, what you put out comes back to you and often times comes back tenfold, so do good deeds.

Conflict

Conflicts, problems or arguments are a part of life and how we deal with them is what it's all about.

In order to overcome a conflict is it better to be at peace or being right? Just because you think your right still does not mean you actually are right. It's all in our perception and we all have different perceptions at different times.

When in the middle of a conflict with a person in our relationship circle is very easy to lose all perspective losing insight to the conflict in question. This can be overcome with practice by creating healthy habits in our relationships. Practice makes perfect or at least it becomes a natural way of our being.

Do your best to keep the conflict conversation on the solution. We often times push each other without thinking causing the conflict to worsen. The conversation will go back and forth on the blame game and the one being blamed will go on the defensive and before you know it things spiral out of control.

Take a deep breath and calmly ask important questions. These questions will help center everyone involved. Questions can be such as what is it going to take to make everyone happy since our relationship is important and worth saving? How can we make each of us happy ending this conflict? With everyone emotional and not being able to see the true perspective can we take a break and talk about this later? How can we resolve this with everyone in the winner's circle?

Problems/conflicts often keep repeating. So many arguments from the repeating conflict. Obviously there are disagreements and most likely a sensitive matter to continue repeating itself. Maybe it's just the way situations are handled and it sets you off the wrong way. Most like it's a difference in our perspectives, character and or morals in turn leads to endless disagreements. Fighting about this will not resolve anything except more fighting. Maybe you just need to agree that you will never agree completely on this issue and agree to disagree.

How can you change your actions in this particular relationship to be supportive? Will one of you or both of you compromise on this issue enough to resolve a win win situation? Last but not least maybe some kind of trade off? Basically what will it take to end happy with your relationship in tact?

By continually having conflict in any relationship you are causing yourself, your life to be out of balance. When one area is off balance it will throw other areas off causing other problems from one conflict without realizing it until eventually something manifests like illness.

Every relationship is different. If you have tried everything in your power to resolve a conflict then maybe you have to walk away. Walking away should be the last thing you do if this relationship is important and worth saving. Maybe you have to be the bigger person and forgive what has happened.

Ask yourself questions like is continuing on with this conflict good for me or anyone? What will become of this relationship if this conflict continues? Will this relationship move forward if not resolved? If your answer to any or all questions is no then simply forgiveness would probably be the best solution.

Forgiveness can restore a person's health along with a huge relief lifted. Remember we are all human and make mistakes. Also, there will always be times you need and want to be forgiven. Do the right thing and forgive often for your health and wellness.

If you have to walk away because maybe this relationship is toxic between you and you both have gone to every resort you can then walk away and forgive as well.

If you don't learn to forgive you will face imbalances in your life in one form or another. It can be the slightest of imbalances, but slight imbalances build into one great big imbalance and before you know it a devastating problem/illness can and often occurs.

Forgiveness de-clutters the mind of unnecessary hurtful emotions like anger, jealousy and resentment just to name a few of these toxic emotions.

Cristie Will

Self-Relationship

None of the Relationships in the end will matter unless you have a healthy relationship with yourself. Without a healthy relationship with yourself you will continue to have other relationship problems, problems with career, problems with money and everything in general. Probably not with all areas, but you will certainly have problems in at least one area of your life and more often than not they will continue just like a circle until corrected.

Do these statements sound familiar? I am stupid, I am not good enough, I am too fat, I am ugly, I am broke, I can't afford that, He/she won't like me, I wished I were, taller, If only I were shorter, I am too young, I am too old, I am not smart enough, I won't win, I can't win? Statements like these or any negative statements to ourselves about ourselves is self-debilitating and causes us to continue in that vicious circle of failure and unhappiness.

When reading these statements can you see why you might be or are stuck? What will it take to change these statements? What else do you need to do to have a healthy relationship with yourself?

Have you ever noticed when you say/mumble something about yourself or to yourself that very thing comes to pass? For example you're late to an appointment and you say repeatedly "I am late and he is going to be so mad!" You walk in the door and he is so mad he unloads. Or the reverse happens and you repeatedly say "I am late, but its ok they are busy!" You walk in and they say something like perfect timing I just finished this last order!

Put this to test and start paying attention to what you are saying and see how it happens just as you speak. Once you test this out and notice this is the case start changing your words to positive words like my examples, but of course change the words to fit your situation. This self-destruction has been going on for years and will take some time to change, so be patient and let time heal all wounds. Continually stop each and every time you mutter a negative remark about yourself and change to a positive remark and as long as you focus on this change then it will start to take effect. You will see a difference in 30 days if you diligently work at it.

Remember if you want change you have to work to change. Every person can change if they choose to. It's by choice that we change or don't change. Our minds are so powerful that we can be, do and become anything we want. The questions are how hard are you willing to work for change? How much do you want change? Are you willing to give it time to take place? If you answered yes then your change is at your doorstep. I am supplying you with examples to say to yourself to help you change the self-destruction talk/chatter we do.

At first it will feel funny replacing the negative talk with positive talk because your mind will tell you that's not true, but keep on and ignore it. Find the phrases that feel right to you such as I am intelligent might feel better and more suiting then saying I am smart.

1. I am smart/intelligent
2. I am love
3. I am beautiful/Handsome
4. I am kind
5. I have what it takes
6. I am grateful
7. I am giving
8. I am deserving
9. I am witty
10. I am fun
11. I am a healer

12. I am sweet
13. I am self-confident
14. I am wise
15. I am at the top of my game
16. I am always on time
17. I am a leader
18. People love me
19. Money flows where I go
20. I have great abundance

Keep it short and simple. Your mind will respond to short and simple phrases faster therefore quicker results. It's easier to say and remember short and simple phrases. You will tend to stick with the program by staying simple. Say these or positive affirmations like these throughout the day and in the evening right before bed. You can also write them to help expedite your process of change. It's really important to speak them and even more powerful in front of the mirror just before bed.

Keep a journal daily to track your progress so you will know if you are actually implementing it. Your journal can be written or digital depending on your preference.

Love Relationships

All relationships need to have love to work. I am going to delve into the relationship area of Spouse, significant other, boyfriend, girlfriend or any intimate relationship to this degree.

In my research I found six areas of love that makes love what love is.

1. Words
2. Looks
3. Time
4. Gifts
5. Action/serve
6. Touch

Words of Love are not just when we say I love you. Love's words are words of encouragement, accomplishments, compliments, and thank you's.

Looks are those looks you get of admiration. The eyes are smiling at you as that are looking you over telling you I am pleased with what I see.

Time is giving of yourself unconditionally to that special love of your life. Whether it's time to go out, to cook, to work in the yard. Spending quality time together.

Gifts can mean giving or receiving anything in the name of love. Could be gifts bought, cards bought or made special for you or your love, or could be a written love note for no reason other than to express love.

Action/Serve is when you help when not asked or when you do something to make your love's life easier.

Cristie Will

Touch is oh those hugs, kisses, touching, holding hands, arms around one another, holding one another, nibbling on their ears or neck and making love.

We are all different and our perceptions are all different as to our view of love. How did we grow up will play into our perceptions. Were our parents loving towards one another, were we loved as children and how much love was given?

Some people are distant and don't like to hug that much while others hug often daily. Neither way is right or wrong. It's just what makes you feel loved is what counts.

To really get the love of your life's attention you just need to pay attention and ask questions. Even if your love doesn't say much their actions will tell you what you need to know.

When you give your love a written love letter watch their facial expressions, their posture, the actions and their words. Did their eyes dance around happily as they read the letter? Were they smiling from ear to ear while reading your letter? Did they touch you with hugs, kisses and if so was it a long hug or kiss? Did they say thank you and how it made them feel?

The same thing will apply if you give your love your time, gifts, hugs, kisses, help them without asking or do something that will make their life easier. By paying attention you will figure out if your love mostly wants your time, or If gifts is what they live for or that love letter is what makes their heart go pitter patter over you. Some don't like gifts they just want your time or hugs or compliments, but by figuring out what they want can often be all you need to have the most loving relationship you can imagine.

It took me years to figure out its right in front of me if I will just take a little time to pay attention I can have an amazing relationship. I did and I will again.

We all want the same thing and that is someone to love and to be loved it's just we all arrive at love in our own way and that's what we have to figure out is the way. Figure out what makes the love of your life feel loved and apply it and what your love life soar.

Remember to make a point to think about them and when you do that it will boomerang back to you and your love will do the same. If you are just starting on implementing this give it 30 days or less to see and feel the results. We are all different, so the results will be different and time frame different for each of us.

Love to you!

4
Careers

Doing What You Love

Do what you love and you will love what you are doing is a true statement. By doing what you love it will not feel like a job and the dread of going to a job you don't like will not be a thought.

Many of us spend hours, days, weeks, months, and many years in careers/jobs that we loath. By being in the wrong career/job is another area that takes a great deal of our time in life, so if this is not right it will cause unbalance in your life. Since we are spiritual beings you can be in a career that is a complete opposition as to where you should be. Another words you are not doing your purpose and your life is constantly struggling in some form from this one issue.

At the end of the day it's finding the work you love and if you can't find that then the next thing would be learn to love the work you have. You could also go into a different career and learn to love that too. Find the balance is what each of us needs to figure out.

To begin with make a list to help you on the path of finding the work you love. Your list needs to contain your strengths, interests and desires. Write down how your assets of strengths, interests and desires could attribute to a career of your dreams. Just let the ideas and list flow, get creative. You have nothing to lose and everything to gain with this exercise.

Once you have finished your list start a goals list. Without goals is like traveling without a map you will just go in circles or all over the map. To get where we want we need a destination and focus....focus....focus.

Once you have written your lists and have finished then do your research. You will not only want to do what you love, but you will want to make a great living at it as well, so the research is crucial.

Now that you are researching check out career options that you desire. Look at how these career paths will interact and shape your long-term goals. Find others working in the field of your choice and ask them for information and support. Check out groups, organizations, and social gatherings to attend to create connections to set yourself up as an expert in your career field. This is important because people want to work with or do business with that they know and feel comfortable. It's who you know to get those great jobs or get your foot in the door to obtain their business.

Finding a new career/job that you love will most likely take some time, so be patient and it will happen. You may have to have different positions or even different companies before finding the perfect fit.

Once you find the career and/or company you want to flourish in ask for projects that interest you to help you soar and find your true happiness with your career. Find a way to express your passion to your boss/employer because this is more often than not the area you will do your best and excel in.

Do your best to stay away from really negative people and be around like minded people. Choose people that are in support of you. 'Birds of a feather flock together', so choose wisely.

To improve in anything it's best to find a way to be able to take constructive feedback to help you with any weaknesses you may have.

If you ever find yourself needing motivation you might give yourself small rewards each time you reach a goal. Make the rewards bigger for bigger projects and so on. Ideas for rewards could be a massage, a manicure/pedicure or a new outfit. Most important do what will make you happy and keep you motivated.

Dress up your workplace/office more soothing for your comfort and uplifting fun look. Put up things to help your motivation like quotes and pictures. Have pictures of your loved ones and things that mean something to you.

If you ever get to the point the job/career is not fulfilling to you anymore and feel it's time to move on then do so. Remember to always put your best foot forward and do the best job possible, because they are still your employer even if you know you are moving on. Always do what's right because you never know if you need to go back to that place of employment, so don't burn any bridges.

If you are contemplating on moving on to a new company, position or career go back to making your lists to narrow down your decisions and get the research underway. This will help you have a better feeling if you should change the path you are on and not wonder if you made the wrong choice. Another words thinking it through from beginning to end of path. Keep at it to find what you love it will always come.

Caring for yourself

I can't stress enough the importance of caring for yourself. You cannot and will not be at your best for others in your life if you neglect yourself. Once you care for yourself you will then be at your best and can care for others within your career and outside of career. By not taking care of yourself you will find things will not get done or you will start to be late or the tardy days will increase and this is just a couple things that will happen. Number one job is care for yourself.

Drink the recommended amount of water daily for you. The rule of thumb has been 64 ounces, eight – 8 ounce glasses. Other professionals say half your body weight, so if you weigh 150 you should drink 75 ounces of water daily. We are all different and one size does not fit all. We do get water from food we eat daily, particularly if eating healthy fruits and veggies, 64 ounces would be good probably. Another thing that would cause you to need more water is strenuous exercise or a job that is very active.

Water helps our bodies remove dangerous chemicals/toxins. Water will rid these toxins and waste from the body through our urination and perspiration along with bowel movements which water aids with constipation to keep those bowels moving. Waste can and does buildup in the body thru dehydration and can cause headaches, toxicity and illness just to name a few health problems. Drinking plenty of water takes the load off of the kidneys and liver by flushing out toxic waste products.

Water also transports valuable nutrients to the body. Blood is approximately 92% water carrying nutrients and oxygen through our bodies. Our Nutrients from the food we eat or supplements are broken down in the digestive system and become water-soluble, so they are dissolved in water. Water helps these nutrients to pass through our body to all the cells and organs. Water also plays a key role in the prevention of disease and illness. So Drink up to your good health caring for yourself.

Caring for yourself with plenty of sleep is of utmost important. By not getting enough sleep this can throw your whole system off. You are more apt to gain weight, be fatigued, foggy thinking and irritability just to name a few.

For a good night's sleep you should be in bed asleep by 10 PM and wake anywhere from 6 AM on, depending on how much sleep you require. Your environment should be quite and be sure to turn off TV's. If you need some soothing music to listen to then go ahead and continue just set a timer so it turns off.

To help you relax and fall asleep sooner you need to incorporate a few minutes of deep breathing. We take shallow breaths and not enough deep breathing. Oxygen is the top priority and we don't do near enough of deep breathing. Without oxygen we would die in a matter of about six minutes. Oxygen helps our bodies remove toxins and that alone will help with our health and wellbeing.

Eating healthy is another must do in caring for yourself. We are all different and will have to come to that happy balance. I can say that all of us need to cut out processed foods. Processed foods are not good for anyone. Processing the food removes all or most nutrients needed by our bodies.

There are so many conflicting articles and books on what to eat and what not to eat. So many diets that it has become mind numbing. Half of your daily intake of food should come from fruits and veggies. Veggies should be more than fruits and watch the fruits because some of them can cause your blood sugar to spike to soon. The other half of your intake should contain protein from nuts, fish, meat, healthy grains, healthy fats and a little dairy like Greek yogurt.

Our soil that we grow our produce in is not as nutrient rich today as in the past, so you should incorporate at least a good multi vitamin daily and Your Omega oils just for insurance along with eating healthy.

Another necessary must for self-care is daily cleanliness such as bathing/showers, caring for your hair/scalp, and teeth/tongue and gums. Our skin is our biggest organ and needs to be cleaned and body brushing regularly. Our bodies rids itself of toxins and other debris through the pours in our skin.

A tongue cleaner is better to use than just brushing your tongue. Brushing your tongue will help get rid of leftover food particles and some bacteria, but not all bacteria will be removed. A tongue cleaner is much better for it will remove deep bacteria deposits and thoroughly stimulates the area cleaning. By cleaning the tongue will also reduce food cravings by removing the leftover food and bacteria. Along with tongue cleaning twice a day you should also brush your teeth and floss after every meal.

Make room for a positive mindset and in order to do this let get of negative self-talk, your limiting beliefs, comparing yourself to others, the need to always be right and resisting change.

In order to have total self-care you need to do everything in some form as I have discussed. Please the rest of the Dots to follow I go into much more depth on all care of yourself and steps to take daily.

Organization and Support

It is so important to be organized at home and at work to make your life easier and smoother. A dis organized home or workplace means you are spending half your time looking for things and that is very nonproductive. Support from family and friends is a big must as well. Without proper support you will continue to hit walls of discouragement from messed up schedules between work and home just to name one wall of disarray.

By being organized you will conserve much energy by being able to find what you need quickly at your fingertips. You can conserve much energy by cutting down going back and forth between tasks. Complete each task before moving on to the next or figure a way to do a couple of tasks at the same time that intertwine with each other.

Since we are all different you need to set up your life organized the way that best works for you. At work you need a filing system that you can find papers or anything quickly and easily. It needs to be set up in such a way that if you need help anyone can go obtain a file for you in a moment's notice.

If possible everything needs a place when you start organizing. Organizing is having a place to put things so if just laying out it will get lost in the shuffle. Now in this electronic day and age we also need to make sure our electronic files are organized as well especially since we have more electronic files then paper files for the most part. Plus do not forget to back up the electronic files regularly. I have and many people have lost important files by not doing this.

A daily checklist is such a must. I use to make fun of my mother having one when I was younger and I now know why she had one. A checklist will improve your life to make things twice as smooth. You cut down on missed appointments, meetings, things being overlooked and making phone calls to grocery shopping just as an example where your life will improve. With this digital age a written or digital checklist works. You want to go the route that you have access at all times since a checklist is basically a way for you to accomplish daily goals.

Set up a calendar written or digital that you can access 24/7 that has work and home schedules together so you can plan and prioritize more efficiently. This will also reduce problems of over or under scheduling, depending on your home and work life. This will also reduce missed appointments and meetings or if a need arises rescheduling when necessary. This will help your home and work life so much smoother and in turn just less problems.

With this digital age and a hurry up life you should set up your phone in a very organized way as well. Make sure you sync your phone with your computer so they go hand in hand and of course back up your phone as well. If you haven't made the leap to a smart phone I would suggest it. You can get all forms of messages, contacts and email plus the phone calls. This way you are in total control and contact and this will help with balancing your life with work and home.

Make sure your home is not only organized as well, but have your working clothes organized and looking good. You can look good on a budget as well. It is well know when you look good and feel good about yourself you will perform better.

Talking to family and friends about your home and work goals will help you stay on track by including them in ways in which they can help. By bringing your family and friends into your home and work goals can help you stay accountable as well.

We are not miracle workers and handle everything every day, so delegate projects when possible at home and at work, depending on your work and home environment. So often we overload ourselves by taking on too much thinking we can do it all and when we do that we not only stress ourselves out this makes room for more errors.

Remember to thank any and all for their help if and when you ask for help. Giving thanks for help will make them feel appreciated and they will want to step up and help when needed. You might even find a way to reward them with small things.

Once you are organized stay on track by making and keeping goals. Your goals need to be daily, weekly, monthly, annually and long term such as 5 and 10 year goals. With goals and holding yourself accountable to them you are apt to accomplish them all and quicker. Goals can be changed because life is every changing. Another step to accomplishing goals is to set time aside to look them over and read them every day to help keep your focus on them. What we focus on is what we have and become in life.

Having trouble reaching goals? Hold yourself accountable. Goals have to be set and made specific, have a support system and have your support to hold you accountable and how they will hold you accountable. Create concrete action items like steps what steps you need to take to lead to your goal. Breakdown each milestone into smaller tasks and give due dates. Set up time with someone in support system or even for yourself and go over to check on where you are on your goals and adjust if necessary. Schedule your time. List the days and times you will devote time to your goal and do not vary unless an emergency.

Goals will help you with organization, so it's a win win with goals.

Income/Financial/Goals

One of the main things pertaining to having a career/job is your income. In order to get to the career/job you love you need to know what your income will be and what you want it to be.

Set a 3 year goal of achieving your desired income level. Goals with action steps will help keep you on track. You need clearly defined and measurable goals. Often times we set to many goals and unrealistic goals. The more you can focus on your goals the better and quicker to obtain them and if you have too many goals you cannot reach them all in a timely manner. Too many goals at once sets yourself up for failure and if you fail then here comes discouragement then we give up.

Set goals that are very specific, realistic and timely. Set two goals at a time and as one drops off set another one. If you have trouble setting goals just start out with one little goal a day and once you reach them every day it gives you the momentum to take off with creative dream goals.

When you are ready to set some goals start with your lists of desires and wants. Then narrow down to two top goals. Ask is this goal Specific enough, realistic and timely? Do these steps on each goal. Check your goals daily to help keep you on track. Write down your goals because the act of writing them down creates thoughts that are real and ideas become concrete. Write out positive outcomes such as work for what you want not what you want to leave behind and if anything is left behind that is a bonus for someone.

If you are having a hard time at any time reaching goals or just keeping your focus I recommend journaling. Writing is such a powerful channel. If you have any blocks sometimes the writing will help you to remove that block. I recommend journaling in the evening because you usually aren't' as rushed and it's before bed. Journaling can help clear your mind as well.

So what does your future hold? Journal about this then write out your long range goals and view this monthly. Write down all the things you want to get done and by when. End of day tomorrow, the end of the week, the end of the month, New Year's Day and year? Do this for one year, two years, 3 years, 5 years, 10 years and 20 years.

If you're not serious about your goals don't waste your time and write them down. Get clear and serious. Make a copy of original goals put them away and in a few years see how many things you have achieved. I say make a copy and put away because it's the original one and your goals you view daily or monthly will change because life is ever changing.

If you have trouble getting clear ideals then take out a sheet of paper and write at the top of the sheet of paper what you want to see manifested, such as my ideal house. Do this for each and every ideal.

Now list all the things that your ideal house must have. Be as specific as possible, the more specific the better. Such as certain appliances, brands, model etc.

Now list all the things your ideal will have. Such as wood floors, carpet and fireplace.

Now list all the things your ideal must not have such as bugs, leaky faucets or roof, needs painting on the outside etc.

Now list all the things that your ideal preferably will not have such as far from work, far from stores and close neighbors.

Make a bucket list this will help with your financial income goals too. Once you know your desires then you will know which path to go for income. Do you need to make more money than thought, about what you thought or less?

Make a list to what your life is right now. List everything about it. What you like, what you don't like, what you want to change, what you must change and what you will change. I know it's a lot of lists and work right now, but it will be easy once you get through this.

The more you can define and get clear about your goals the more you will reach them. This will cause you to set more goals and it's a chain reaction. When first starting out it is a little harder because it's new and worthwhile. Anything worthwhile will take some work.

Financial goals will dramatically improve your life because that is what most of us want in life. While money can't buy happiness it can sure make the ride in life a little smoother.

If you make goals a habit you will have a purpose all your life and everyone wants a purpose, so what's your purpose?

5
Spirituality and Balance

Connecting and Finding your Spirituality

My spirituality was the biggest void missing in my life, so I cannot express enough that finding this connecting Dot is number one. I knew it in my heart all along, but it just didn't hit me until I saw The Daniel Plan on the web. I clicked on The Daniel Plan and I could feel God's power go through every cell of my body and I knew this was my missing piece.

I found once I connected back with my Creator, God, then everything else in my life started to flow and finding real peace. It helped me to forgive myself for all the pain and hurt I had done to others as well as myself. It helped me forgive others that hurt me over the years as well. One thing lead to another then real gratitude and contentment came about. I have all that I need in life because my creator always provides a way to have everything I need. Is life perfect? No, that's in the next life.

I was lost for the last 20 years because I walked away from my Creator. I was naive but didn't realize it at the time. I walked away from God after my first husband molested my daughter. I just didn't understand how I could meet a good man in church and he do such an injustice. What I now realize is we are all human and make mistakes. Some mistakes are life changing, but will work out the best in the end. Even though the horrible injustice that my first husband caused I did have two beautiful children that I am thankful for.

I now realize that as long as I am alive I will see blessing after blessing, but will have set backs or injustices from time to time and that is part of life. I will not walk away from my Creator again.

The Daniel Plan lit me up on my way. Also, I read the book The Dynamic Laws of Prosperity by Catherine Ponder which helped me so much. I bought this book about a year ago and suddenly every time I walked by the bookshelf it was calling out to me to read. God was telling me to read this book I could just feel it, so I read it and it was absolutely a very valuable tool. I don't think I would have picked this book back up if it weren't for The Daniel Plan being the spark that lit me up. I now read all the spiritual self-help along with my bible for more understandings.

As I started implementing some of the suggestions, such as decree's and affirmations from Catherine Ponders book I noticed things changing, such as clarity on what I wanted. Other times when I needed something it would just appear by either someone offering what I needed or suddenly I would come across an opportunity to make the money I needed to obtain it.

I have tried different things over the years that didn't work, but it's because I didn't stick with it long enough or it was because it wasn't for me. If it's for you then you have to have the patience to stay with it the whole way. The mistake many people and myself have made over the years is stopping just shy of our goals to come to fruition.
I found by listening to my own gut instinct and following it, I don't make mistakes when I truly listen and follow what my creator is telling me. At first it was hard to follow my gut instinct because I wanted to do what I thought was right and by doing what I wanted to is when I realized that is why I am making all these mistakes. The more I listen to what I am supposed to do the easier it gets. It has now become automatic listening to my Creator on what to do.

We all are at where we are today because of our choices to go down the paths we have taken. We have the choice to choose a different path at any time you just have to have the will to do so. Remember it's never too late unless your time has expired on this earth.

Cristie Will

I put the brakes on to quit mindlessly going through life with no purpose which we all should do. We all have a purpose, so please stop to smell the roses to allow the purpose to come forth. When you find your purpose that is when your tranquility will set in and take you to new heights that you never dreamed possible.
I have a story to tell so that I can help others. I went through everything I have been through in order to help others. Eventually we end up where we are supposed to. You can take the right paths to get there and make it a much easier ride to your destination. The reason we have more struggles then necessary is because of taking the wrong path. The wrong path is just a detour to where you will end up, but the wrong path is what throws those obstacles and extra problems in your way.

Everyone has their own story to tell that will help others. I encourage everyone to reach out and help others. Life is easier with others, so set out to make your life an easier fun journey.

We are all different and you have to find your own spirituality, your creator, your higher self or whatever that may be for you. If you are not sure then just explore and you will find your spirituality.

Our creator has given us all the answers we need. To get to the answers needed just ask yourself questions until the answer comes and it will come. Start out with the question what is it that I really want? Make a list of what you want and a list of what you don't want. Take your time it could take you a few days to really get to the bottom of the list. Once you have the list it may give you the answer or it may narrow it down and you have to ask more questions, but stay at it because the answer will come.

Thank you for reading my book. By reading my book you are looking for a change to better your life and you have the power to do that.

Deep Breathing

Deep breathing has so many benefits that a whole book could be written about it. I am going to list the main benefits for you now. Deep Breathing is free, you don't have to buy anything, and always with you. Also, it's convenient and don't have to buy any clothing or equipment either.

1. Speeds up your metabolism increasing ability to lose weight faster
2. Normalizes your body chemistry
3. Gives you glowing skin
4. Provides mental clarity
5. Increased your energy
6. Harmony with Mind Body
7. Reduces stress
8. Raises Self Esteem
9. Mood Booster
10. Heightens Athletic Performance

The top ten reasons for deep breathing are enough we should all be doing it, but we aren't. We think oh that's too much trouble or I don't have time. These are excuses and how I know is they were my excuses. You do have time and it's no trouble. It's like everything once you start doing it and doing it long enough it will be a habit.

Having time is easy. Take a five minute break at work and breath. If you can and want to take longer like the 15 minutes that we normally get with work then do that. Take five minutes when you awake in the morning, go to sleep at night or better yet take five minutes in the morning and in the evening. We waste that much time easily during the day, so take that wasted time and make it productive to good health and well-being.

No trouble at all. Have you ever started something new and it be smooth sailing like you have been doing it for years? Of course you haven't. You may have done things that feel right and you are supposed to do it, but it's still a learning curve. Well the very same thing is for deep breathing a learning curve. Once you get this down it will be second nature and you won't even realize you are doing it. It's quite simply magical.

Wanting to speed up that metabolism to lose weight and not gain back so easily? You can do just that with Deep Breathing. Deep Breathing raises your metabolism causing you to lose weight and at the same time balances your body chemistry causing you to have that normal metabolism you were born with. Yes you can cause your metabolism to go even higher with exercise and other metabolism boosting foods too. There is a study out there that says 73% of people that need to lose weight have underperforming metabolisms. This does make sense. Save money on beauty products and get the glowing skin by just deep breathing everyday regularly. Of course the more time and the more often you do the deep breathing the quicker and longer lasting your results will be.

Do you have fog brain? Do you want to start a project that you need that crisp mental clarity? Lift the brain fog and gain the crisp mental clarity just by deep breathing.

Who doesn't want more energy? Deep breathing gives you more energy. With more energy comes more accomplishments along with the feeling of vitality. In turn brings harmony between your mind and body. We all know your mind and body has to have the balance to be healthy.

So many illness's today are brought on by stress, so you can cut down on stress, doctor visits, and missing work just by doing deep breathing.

Deep breathing raises your self-esteem because you feel better. Deep breathing nourishes every cell in our bodies and by doing that it causes your mood to lift and with a lifted mood you feel good and your self-esteem goes up.

Want to heighten you athletic ability? Deep breathing can take you to that next level and in time take you to the top of your game. The biggest thing is to start and do it regularly. Start the deep breathing and no matter what you do not have to miss it or shouldn't.

I can write about this because it helped me with every one of these issues, so I am living proof. I was searching on ways to feel better and lose weight and came across several books that helped me understand deep breathing, so I took the advice and it does work.

For you to further your knowledge and understanding of deep breathing do your research and most importantly start the deep breathing on yourself. You will see and feel the difference and not only that, if you don't see or feel any difference it cost you nothing.

To help you with your research I would suggest you to obtain Pam Grout's book called Jumpstart your Metabolism. You can either purchase it or check it out at the library. Other books that explain breathing are Yoga Books. Browse through the book store, library or online for Yoga books and do your research that way. Of course you can just type deep breathing into your internet search engine and go from there.

Please don't wait on the deep breathing since it's so vital and the health benefits outweigh any reason not to. Take a deep breath literally.

Cristie Will

Affirmations that Make It

For positive lasting changes affirmations need to be spoken and written. If you want to go the extra distance to make even quicker changes you can record your voice speaking to you and you listen to them when you can and at night when you go to sleep.

Here's what I found with Affirmations that I don't think I have read anywhere else and that is start out with a fast start, but don't overload with too many. If you start out with too many you will get burnt out and not do them at all. Affirmations do work and I want you to see the fruits of your labor, so please keep it to no more than 3 affirmations. Short sweet and simple. The 3 affirmations to start out with need to be towards one goal such as losing weight or whatever that goal may be.

Always speak and write out the affirmations as if it has already happened. Your mind does not know the difference, but your mind will put off your goals if you keep saying things like I will lose this weight or I will get that new car. Yes you will lose that weight and you will get that new car, but when next year, ten years? See your mind has that new car in mind, but it doesn't know when you want it.

I have read where it says to state your affirmations I lost all my excess weight or I, Cristie Will, lost all my excess weight. I felt like if I say I, Cristie Will, lost all my excess weight then I had both ways covered, so that is the way I state my affirmations and they do work.

Affirmations only work if you work them. Affirmations are not the only thing you need to do to get the end result. Affirmations help you get the end result but It's only one of the dots to your end result.
The reason why affirmations are so powerful is because how you arrived at being who you are is through your words, thoughts and actions. Words become thoughts and thoughts become things and things

become actions and combined is each of us. Purposefully speaking and writing your new life is just that. Speaking and writing your way to create your new life.

First off you need to be clear on what you want and which of your goals you want to reach first. Then find 10 15 affirmations you think will work and write them out then speak them out. Look in the mirror and speak them. Figure out which 3 feel right and most comfortable to you. Do they flow off the tongue and out of your pen onto paper? If the answer is yes then you found your 3 affirmations. If not then keep going. Maybe your found 2 of the 3 and the others on the list just don't feel right then keep searching for more and get the right one.

Affirmations are strong and a great tool to help you get to your goal quicker, but if you don't use the right affirmations and do not use them consistently you will take much longer and you may not get the exact results you're looking for. With the right affirmations you will get the results you are looking for and quicker results providing you use them daily and more often.

Affirmation Examples below:

Goals:
    I choose to set goals, and work to achieve them.
    When I set a goal I reach and nothing can stop me.
    I stay with my goals until accomplished.

Weight loss:
    I live best when I eat less.
    I eat only nourishing foods for my Mind, Body and soul.
    I feel great at my perfect weight of 120 (fill in the weight you want to weigh)

Cristie Will

Self-Esteem:
> I love myself more and more every day in every way.
> I care about my wellbeing and take care of myself.
> I love everything about me.

Exercise:
> When I exercise I feel great.
> I enjoy exercising
> I choose to exercise regularly

Prosperity:
> I am a money magnet and money flows freely to me.
> Infinite riches are now freely flowing into my life.
> It's okay for me to have everything I want.

Health:
> I am healthier today and every day.
> I choose to be healthy and it shows.
> I am vibrantly healthy and radiantly beautiful.

Relationships:
> I now give and receive love freely,
> I am now attracting my perfect soul mate.
> I love to love and be loved.

Happiness:
> I feel happy and blissful every day.
> Happiness follows me everywhere I go.
> I only see and attract happiness.

Meditation

There are many ways for Meditation. Breathing can be and is part of meditation, but more to it than breathing. Especially if your only focus is to breath oxygen into your cells for health reasons only.

Meditation can be prayer/chanting, breathing, exercise or listening to music or just sitting outdoors viewing the beauty of it all.

You can start out just meditating a couple of minutes a day building to 30 minutes or more. You choose what works best for you. The goal of meditating is to allow your mind to rest from thoughts passing through and just letting them pass without taking care of each thought.

To start your meditation you need a quite comfortable spot. Concentrate on breathing at first, the inhalation and exhalation and once relaxed just lie there or set there, depending on if you are laying down or sitting up in a comfortable chair.

There is no right or wrong way to meditate. In the beginning you may be uncomfortable and feel silly, but that's ok and normal. It may be difficult feeling at first because your focus drifts since your mind is probably racing around.

It's best to meditate first thing in the morning to be able to tap into your inner conscious easier plus less distractions first thing in the morning. It's also good to meditate just before going to bed to help you relax for a good night's rest, but also to tap into your inner conscious.

After you have strengthened your meditation practices and feel comfortable then experiment at other times, like at your desk before a long meeting or starting that big project, after a workout and anytime in between.

Meditation works best when practiced daily, so start simple but stay regular, such as doing your meditation at the same time every day for the same duration. It's best to really start out with 5 minutes, but 3 minutes is ok for beginners and do that daily. Then meditate 20 minutes once a week, but the same time and day of the week for the 20 minute mediation as well. Seasoned meditators recommend 20 minutes daily twice a day and I must admit that is what I do as well. I think it's great if you can work up to 20 minutes a day twice a day, but start out slow so you don't overwhelm yourself making you stop altogether.

You don't have to, but it's a good idea to stretch out and loosen your body before sitting or lying down for meditating.

As you are in position repeat a mantra, this is not necessary, but does help quiet the mind. A mantra is repeating a sound, phrase or word over and over until you silence your mind and enter the meditative state. The mantra can be anything you choose, as long as it's simple and easy to remember such as, one um, om, calm, love and peace are a few good easy ones.

Meditation will help you to slow your mind down from this fast paced world we live in and allow your intuition to show itself much more strongly in turn allowing you to align you with your intentions.

Putting music on really low in the background really helps me to. Find music made for mediation. It needs to be low and soothing, just instrumental. Music or sounds like water is also soothing and helps as long as it's subtle, down low. We are all different, so do whatever it takes and feels right for you.

In addition to mental, emotional and physical health benefits meditation may help with the following and much more:

Allergies
Anxiety Disorders
Asthma
Binge Eating
Cravings/Food Addiction
Depression
Fatigue
Heart Disease
High Blood Pressure
Chronic Pain
Sleep Problems
Substance/Drug Abuse

Since meditation not only pertains to meditating but to breathing as well it's no wonder it has so many health benefits. Meditation is a journey for each of us and is different for all of us. The whole purpose is to calm the mind while achieving inner peace and going on to a higher spiritual place. It is important to know it could take years of practice to achieve the level of awareness like the pros in meditation, but it doesn't matter. Meditation being a journey is like climbing a mountain where each and every step brings you closer to the top.

The main thing is just to start meditating and don't be a bit concerned with the quality of the meditation. Just as long as you feel calmer and more at peace by the end of the practice and you will know that your meditation was successful if you accomplished the peace and calmness that you should experience.

Cristie Will

Quick Steps for Meditation:

Choose quite place, Wear comfy clothes, Decide how long, Stretch out, Sit or lie in comfortable position, and Close your eyes.

Visualization

I cannot stress enough how important visualization is. Visualization is so important since our minds work with pictures and not words.

If you can see it in your mind then you can achieve it outwardly. There is no limit what you can achieve with Visualization. Along with visualization takes action to achieve, but by visualizing the action is natural and your mind will work you towards the action. It's like a domino effect. One domino touches one and then the next and the next began to fall and everything falls into place.

The visualization was difficult at first, but it got easier each day.

6
Processed Foods, Healthy Eating & Detoxing

Processed Foods

Processed foods are just what it says, its food that has been taken apart and so many chemicals added that it is no longer nourishment. Food is supposed to be for our nourishment. With all the processed stuff along with our high paced lifestyles it's no wonder obesity and diseases of all kinds have skyrocketed to an all-time high. The only real way to put a stop to it is do not buy this crap.

We cannot rely on our government to protect us. If you read what is going on in this world with the GMO's you will see other countries are banning them left and right, but our government is just allowing it all day long. Most of these fast food restaurants in other countries can't load their food up with all these chemicals, because the country has said no and we should too say no.

A surprising new food source could be causing you stomach irritation. Your body can be treating genetically modified corn sources as a toxin. If you think that you may have a corn sensitivity, this list of corn aliases below can help you eliminate it from your diet. This is probably not all the sources since they change often.

Alpha tocopherol	Polenta
Ascorbic acid	Polydextrose Sorbitol
Baking powder	Starch
Calcium stearate	Sucrose
Caramel	Treacle
Cellulose	Vanilla extract
Citric acid	Xanthan gum
Corn flour	Xylitol

Corn oil	Zein
Cornmeal	Dextrin
Cornstarch	Dextrose (glucose)
Corn syrup	Distilled White Vinegar
Diglycerides	Gluten (corn gluten)
Ethylene	Golden Syrup
Ethyl acetate	High fructose corn syrup
Ethyl lactate	Inositol PolydextroseSorbitol
Fibersol-2	Invert Sugar
Fructose	Malt
Fumaric acid	Malodetrin
Monosodium glutamate (MSG)	Margarine
Monoglycerides	

List of Names for Artificial Sweeteners. Replacing sugar with artificial sweeteners may be doing your body more harm than good. This list will help you avoid these dangerous chemicals.

ACK	APM
Ace K	AminoSweet (but not in US)
Equal Spoonful (also +aspartame)	Aspartyl-phenylalanine-1-methyl
ester	Sucaryl
Sweet One	Canderel (not in US)
Sunett	NatraTaste Blue
Licorice	Equal Classic
NutraSweet	
TwinSweet (Europe only)	
Calcium cyclamate	
Cologran	
Sugar alcohol	
Sugar alcohol (from glucose and sorbitol)	

Artificial Sweeteners continued

Rebiana	Natrulose
Sugar alcohol	Sugar alcohol
Zerose	Acid saccharin
ZSweet	Equal Saccharin
Glycerin	Maltitol Syrup & Powder
Glycerine	Hydrogenated Maltose

Hydrogenated High Maltose Glucose Syrup

Trichlorogalactosucrose	Trichlorosucrose
Necta Sweet	Equal Sucralose
Sodium Saccharin	NatraTaste Gold
Sweet N Low	Splenda
Sweet Twin	

Dangerous Food Additives

This is just a list of many chemicals/toxins/preservatives/additives on the market and they change periodically.

102 & E102 Tartrazine (food color)
104 & E104 Quinoline Yellow (food color)
107 & E107 Yellow 2G (food color)
110 & E110 Sunset Yellow (Yellow food color #6)
120 & E120 Carmines, Cochineal (food color)
122 & E122 Azorubine, Carmoisine (food color)
123 & E123 Amaranth (Red food color #2)
124 & E124 Ponceau, Brilliant Scarlet (food color)
127 & E127 Erythrosine (Red food color #2)
E128 Red 2G (Red food color)
129 & E129 Allura Red AC (food color)
E131 Patent Blue (food color)
132 & E132 Indigotine, Indigo Carmine (food color)

Dangerous Food Additives Continued

133 & E133 Brilliant Blue (food color)
142 & E142 Acid Brilliant Green, Green S, Food Green (food color)
143 Fast Green (food color)
150 & E150 Caramel (food color)
151 & E151 Activated Vegetable Carbons, Brilliant Black (food color)
154 Food Brown, Kipper Brown, Brown FK (food color)
155 & E155 Chocolate Brown HT, Brown HT (food color)
160b & E160b Bixin, Norbixin, Annatto Extracts E173 Aluminium (preservatives)
E180 Latol Rubine, Pigment Rubine (preservatives)

200 & E200-203 Potassium & Calcium Sorbates ,Sorbic Acid (preservatives)
210 & E210 Benzoic Acid (preservatives)
211 & E211 Sodium Benzoate (preservatives)
212 & E212 Potassium Benzoate (preservatives)
213 & E213 Calcium Benzoate (preservatives)
E214 Ethyl Para Hydroxybenzonate (preservatives)
E215 Sodium Ethyl Para Hydroxybenzonate (preservatives)
216 & E216 Propyl P Hydroxybenzonate, Propylparaben (preservatives)
E217 Sodium Propyl P Hydroxybenzonate (preservatives)
220 & E220 Sulphur Dioxide (preservatives)
221 & E221 Sodium Sulphite (preservatives)
222 Sodium Bisulphite (preservatives)
223 & E223 Sodium Metabisulphite (preservatives)
224 & E224 Potassium Metabisulfite (preservatives)
225 & E225 Potassium Sulfite (preservatives)
E226 Calcium Sulphite (preservatives)
E227 Calcium Hydrogen Sulphite (preservatives)
E228 Potassium Bisulphite, Potassium Hydrogen Sulphite (preservatives)
E230 Diphenyl, Biphenyl (preservatives)

Dangerous Food Additives Continued

E231 Orthophenyl Phenol (preservatives)

E236 Formic Acid (preservative)

E239 Hexamine, Hexamethylene Tetramine (preservatives)

249 & E249 Potassium Nitrate (preservative)

250 & E250 Sodium Nitrite (preservative)

251 & E251 Sodium Nitrate (preservative)

252 & E252 Potassium Nitrate (preservative)

260 & E260 Acetic Acid, Glacial (preservatives)

280 to 283 Calcium or Potassium or Sodium Propionates, Propionic Acid

310 & E310 Propyl Gallate (Synthetic Antioxidant)

311 & E311 Octyl Gallate (Synthetic Antioxidant)

312 & E312 Dodecyl Gallate (Synthetic Antioxidant)

319 & E319 TBHQ, Tert Butylhydroquinone (Synthetic Antioxidants)

320 & E320 Butylated Hydroxyanisole (BHA) (Synthetic Antioxidants)

321 & E321 Butylated Hydroxytoluene (BHT) or Butylhydroxytoluene

407 & E407 Carrageenan (Thickening & Stabilizing Agent)

413 & E413 Tragacanth (thickener & Emulsifier)

414 & E414 Acacia Gum (Food Stabilizer)

416 Karaya Gum (Laxative, Food Thickener & Emulsifier)

421 & E421 Mannitol (Artificial Sweetener)

430 Polyxyethylene Stearate (Emulsifier)

431 Polyxyl Stearate (Emulsifier)

E432 - E435 Polyoxyethylene Sorbitan Monostearate

433 - 436 Polysorbate (Emulsifiers)

441 & E441 Gelatine (Food Gelling Agent)

466 Sodium CarboxyMethyl Cellulose

507 & E507 Hydrochloric Acid (Hydrolyzing Enhancer & Gelatin Production)

518 & E518 Magnesium Sulphate (Tofu Coagulant)

536 & E536 Potassium Ferrocyanide (Anti Caking Agent)

Dangerous Food Additives Continued

553 & E553 & E553b Talc (Anti Caking, Filling, Softener, Agent)

620 - 625 MSG Monosodium Glutamate, Glutamic Acid, all Glutamates (Flavor Enhancers)
627 & E627 Disodium Guanylate (Flavor Enhancers)
631 & E631 Disodium Inosinate 5 (Flavor Enhancers)
635 & E635 Disodium Ribonucleotides 5 (Flavor Enhancers)

903 & E903 Camauba Wax (used in Chewing Gums, Coating and Glazing
905 & 905 a,b,c Paraffin, Vaseline, White Mineral Oil (Solvents, Coating, Glazing, Anti
Foaming, Lubricant Agents in Chewing Gums)
924 & E924 Potassium Bromate (Agent used in Bleaching Flour)
925 & E925 Chlorine (Agent used in Bleaching Flour, Bread Enhancer and Stabiliser)
926 Chlorine Dioxide (Bleaching Flour and Preservative Agent)
928 & E928 Benzoyl Peroxide (Bleaching Flour and Bread enhancer Agent)
950 & E950 Potassium Acesulphame (Sweetener)
951 Aspartame (Sweetener)
952 & E952 Cyclamate and Cyclamic Acid (Sweeteners)
954 & E954 Saccharine (Sweetener)

1202 & E1202 Insoluble Polyvinylpyrrolidone Insoluble (Stabiliser and Clarifying Agent added to Wine, Beer, Pharmaceuticals)

1403 Bleached Starch (Thickenner and Stabiliser)

MSG (Monosodium Glutamate): Another silent killer

Did you know that MSG is worse for your health than alcohol, nicotine and other drugs that is probably in your kitchen cabinets right this minute?

MSG (Monosodium Glutamate) is a well-known flavor enhancer that's mostly known for widely use to Chinese food, but is added to thousands of the foods most of us eat regularly, especially processed foods or in a majority of restaurants.

MSG is one of the worst food additives on the market and is even used in Baby food and baby formula.

Many of the adverse effects linked to regular use of MSG including, but not limited to:

Obesity, Eye Damage, Headaches, Fatigue/disorientation and depression just to name a few.

Short term reactions known as MSG Symptom Complex can involve symptoms such as the following:

Numbness, burning sensation, tingling, facial pressure, tightness, chest pain, difficult breathing, headache, nausea, rapid heartbeat, Drowsiness and weakness.

List of ingredients that Always have MSG:

Autolyzed Yeast	Calcium Caseinate	Gelatin
Glutamate	Glutamic Acid	Hydrolyzed Protein
Monopotassium Glutamate	Monosodium Glutamate	Sodium Caseinate
Testured Protein	Yeast Extract	
Yeast Nutrient	Yeast Food	

List of ingredients that often contain MSG or can create MSG during processing:

Flavors and Flavorings Flavorings	Seasonings	Natural Flavors and
Natural Chicken Flavoring	Soy Sauce	Soy Protein Isolate
Stock	Broth	Malt Extract
Enzyme Modified	Carrageenan	Maltodetrin
Protease	Corn Starch	Citric Acid
Anything Pasteurized	Natural Pork Flavor	Natural Beef Flavoring
Soy Protein	Bouillon	Malt Flavoring
Pectin	Enzymes	Powdered Milk
Anything Protein Fortified		

It does take a bit more planning and learning to be MSG free, but well worth it to rid yourself and your family of these risks. I say it's better to be safe than sorry.

Another good rule of thumb that makes shopping easier is if the products you are looking to buy have more than 5 ingredients other than real food it's probably has something bad in it.

Eating out you can ask your waiter for a list of menu items without MSG and request that no MSG be added to your meal, but the only place you can be certain of no MSG is your own kitchen.

The chemicals, toxins, preservatives are bombarding us daily and we cannot live in this society without being exposed to some of them. What we can do is avoid as much as possible and regularly detox the rest out of our systems as often as possible. The sad truth this is only some of them. There is so much more out there and in order to give you more I would have to write a whole book on them. The worst of it is the Manufacturers change the names of these additives and know how to do it to skirt under the law.
 Here are a few tips to help you.

1. Stay away from processed meats like bacon, hot dogs, Bologna and sausage just to name a few. Sodium nitrate accounts for the appetizing red hue, but this additive is so bad it can lead to cancer and other ailments.

2. Stick to low-mercury fish such as American-farmed tilapia instead of swordfish or tuna since overexposure of mercury can cause memory problems, fatigue, and untold other health issues, but Choose the farmed fish carefully. Studies have shown that some farm-raised fish contain more polychlorinated biphenyl and over ten times the amount of dioxin.

3. Cut way back on canned goods, unless you can foods yourself. Cans are commonly lined with bisphenol-A, an organic compound that may be associated with diabetes and heart disease among other health issues.

4. Cut back on meat and dairy products. These animal products could still have harmful contaminants like polybrominated diphenyl ethers, polychlorinated biphenyl and dioxins. Even though many of these toxins have been banned, they could still be present in our soil.

5. Stop using artificial sweeteners that are in a vast array of products such as diet soda just to name one. Prolonged exposure to aspartame can lead to nerve cell damage, dizziness, headaches and other ailments. This has been shown in studies like giving rat's brain tumors.

6. Choose organic chicken. It has been discovered that there are traces of arsenic in non-organic chickens. This dangerous chemical can lead to cancer, diabetes and heart disease. Plus another study found different antibiotic-resistant bacteria in non-organic chicken and poultry.

7. Only purchase milk that says "no RBGH" on the packaging since recombinant bovine growth hormone has been linked with breast cancer. To avoid this all together drink unsweetened, nut or rice milk.

8. Manufactured snacks are loaded with hydrogenated oils to lengthen the shelf life of
products which are linked to diabetes and heart disease. It doesn't stop there they are also loaded with salt, corn syrup and other unhealthy ingredients.

9. Stay away from artificially-colored foods. The list is too long to name on the artificially colored foods, so just read the label and if it's in the product don't buy it. Studies show that blue 1 and 2, red 3 and yellow 6 suffered from brain, adrenal gland, thyroid, and kidney tumors. This is just the beginning of what all this can do to us.

10. Always buy organic produce. Lingering pesticides can lead to nervous and reproductive system damage, not to mention cancer. GMO's (genetically Modified Organism's) are shown to cause a multitude of problems as well.

11. Use stainless steel or cast iron cookware to prepare your meals just like back in the days before Teflon. Teflon releases gases when exposed to high temperatures, which puts you at risk for heart disease among other health issues.

12. You should never microwave food in plastic. Exposure to heat can cause the bisphenol-A found in plastics to break down and potentially contaminate your food and you should not put in dishwasher because of the high heat, so hand wash your plastic ware to be safe.

Effects of Water

Our bodies are made up of around 60 to 75% water. It is no surprise that we need water and the fact drinking to little or too much water can cause health issues. Too much water could cause mineral imbalances and too little water could cause dehydration, headaches and fatigue among other issues.

The general rule of thumb is 64 ounces of water daily. Some professionals say half your body weight in ounces of water per day while others say men should drink about 3 liters (13 cups) and women need to drink about 2.2 liters (9 cups) of water per day. We are all different and need to take into account various factors as to what each of us require from day to day. An example to consider would be the water content of fresh fruits and vegetables may increase hydration in the body.

Water should be increased during hot or humid temperatures, high altitudes of 8,200 feet and above, during exercise, illness/fever, diarrhea and vomiting, infections of the bladder or urinary tract, pregnancy, breast feeding and increased during alcohol intake.

There are different types of water such as tap, bottled, filtered, distilled, and alkaline ionized water. The type of water a person chooses mostly depends on cost and availability, as not everybody has access to the best sources of water.

Tap water is the most readily available, but depending where your tap water is from may not be the best safest option. Some cities/towns have very good water purification systems while others don't. It's a good idea to research your city/towns purification system to see if it warrants a home purification system in your home.

Water Filters can help remove toxins that can pose a threat to your water, but you should know what toxins are in your water in order to choose the right filter.

Distillation is boiling water to remove impurities and toxins. Some think the naturally occurring minerals in non-distilled water are beneficial to health and could be.

Bottle water is popular, portable and handy. It's great for people without access to safe drinking water. There is growing concern about the chemicals from the plastic seeping into the water and concerns with the increasing numbers of bottles filling the landfills.

Water Ionizers are gaining much more recognition on the ability to create alkaline water through electrolysis which may have benefits since our bodies are healthiest slightly alkalized.

Water can raise your metabolism as much as three percent. If you are dehydrated that can mimic hunger and cause food cravings. Water can prevent and cure many of our illnesses such as high blood pressure, gallbladder stones, skin problems, osteoporosis, heart disease, asthma, allergies, colon health, coughs, colds, gout, hemorrhoids, diabetes, arthritis, lung conditions, insomnia, kidney stones and hepatitis.

There is a growing concern about potential links between an array of health issues including cancer and chemicals found in drinking water. Whether you drink tap water or well water, additives and contaminates linked to cancer probably exist in your water. Here are a few of the chemicals found in our water supply and there are many others.

Antimony is a metal found in natural deposits as ores containing other elements. The most widely used antimony compound is antimony trioxide, which is used as a flame retardant.

Asbestos is a fibrous mineral occurring in natural deposits. Because asbestos fibers are resistant to heat and most chemicals and have been mined for use in products such as roofing materials, brake pads, and cement pipe often used in distributing water to communities.

Arsenic may be found in water which has flowed through arsenic-rich rocks. Severe health effects have been observed in populations drinking arsenic-rich water over long periods in countries around the world.

Barium is a lustrous, machinable metal which exists in nature only in ores containing mixtures of elements. In particular, it is used in well drilling operations where it is directly released into the ground where can seep into our water.

Beryllium is a metal found in natural deposits as ores containing other elements, and in some precious stones. Probably the biggest use is in making metal alloys for nuclear reactors and the aerospace industry.

Cadmium is a metal found in natural deposits as ores containing other elements. The greatest use of cadmium is primarily for metal plating and coating operations.

Chromium is a metal found in natural deposits as ores containing other elements. The greatest use of chromium is in metal alloys such as stainless steel and protective coatings.

Lead is a metal found in natural deposits as ores containing other elements. It is often used in household plumbing materials and water service lines used to bring water from the main to the home.

Mercury is a liquid metal found in natural deposits as ores containing other elements. Products such as batteries, fluorescent light bulbs, switches, and other control equipment account for 50% of mercury used.

Food Preparation & Storage

One of the biggest things to help with eating healthy and sticking to a weight loss program is food preparation and storage. I know in the past if I didn't have meals and snacks readily available then I would grab the first unhealthy food like chips or candy. Now that I decided to prepare ahead of time it has made all the difference in the world. When I get hungry I can grab healthy food now and stay with the program of a healthy lifestyle.

The first must do is clean your home of all the bad toxic foods and food products.

1.   Take a list of toxins found in foods and start with your pantry and toss
2.   Take that same list once finished with pantry and clean refrigerator/freezer of toxic foods.

To do list for food preparation & storage:

1.   Plan your meals for the week.
2.   Check your pantry, freezer and Refrigerator for items on hand
3.   Make a grocery shopping list
4   Make trip to the grocery store for needed items

Now that you have all the things you need to prepare for healthy eating you will start cooking and getting fresh veggies ready to grab for snacking.

I always keep celery and carrots on hand for snacking, putting in salads and cooking. First off I take my celery and the both ends off. I generally cut off ½ inch on top and about an inch of the base of the celery bunch. Wash thoroughly and cut in half or and place in dish with lid and fill with water placing into refrigerator. I do the same thing with my carrots. By doing this they have a longer shelf life and they are readily available.
I buy salad mixtures bring home, wash and place in a container with a lid that helps preserves fresh veggies and fruits longer. These containers do work and I suggest getting them. They have different varieties available. They are plastic and there are concerns about the plastic. Just make sure they are BPA free and you don't heat in them. I have several different sizes of these containers and cut up other veggies in them as well. By doing this I have fresh veggies for 7 to 10 days and if I don't do this then it's 3 to 4 days and my fruit and veggies seem to go bad. The containers I have found have a green lid with clear container or green lid and green container. I don't have a preference on brand.

Always buy organic when possible. Below is a list of fruits and veggies that separate what must be organic and what is ok as non-organic.

These need to be organic:	These do not have to be organic:
• Apples	Avocados
• Strawberries	Sweet Corn
• Grapes	Pineapples
• Celery	Cabbage
• Peaches	Sweet peas (frozen)
• Spinach	Onions
• Sweet bell peppers	Asparagus
• Nectarines (imported)	Mangoes
• Cucumbers	Papayas
• Cherry tomatoes	Kiwi
• Snap peas (imported)	Eggplant
• Potatoes	Grapefruit
• Hot peppers	Cantaloupe (domestic)
• Blueberries (domestic)	Cauliflower
• Zucchini	Sweet potatoes

Keep in mind this list of items can change. Some of the ok organic items could get to the point where they are grown without all the pesticides and/or GMO's become banned. The list could also change such as the do not have to be organic need to be organic simply because they are now using pesticides or they have become GMO. With the ever changing world it's best to stay abreast of our foods.

I will cook up a pot of rice, preferably black rice since it's better for you, then I dish up in some one serving size containers or bigger containers for more than one person and freeze these. Also, I do the same thing for Beans like lentils, black beans and other beans. Dish the beans in containers and freeze.

Another great food to prepare is cauliflower if you rice it for say cauliflower potatoes or want to make a pizza crust or even use as rice instead of actual rice. Place your cauliflower into a food processer and rice it quickly and place in storage containers or freezer bags and freeze. If you don't have a food processor you can even cup up finely by hand or you can follow the instructions on your blender and rice it as well this too just takes a bit longer.

I drink smoothies often in the morning or even at lunch, so I will bag up most of my ingredients in freezer bags and freeze such as kale, celery, cucumber, berries, bananas, apples and pineapple or whatever you choose. I will take ice cube trays with lids and freeze plain unsweetened yogurt and different nut milks separately. This way you can toss in some yogurt or nut milks for your smoothies and other dishes like ice-cream. You can even freeze dairy milk if you drink that.

For that sweet tooth I will slice and keep frozen bananas in my freezer to make ice cream and many different desserts.

I will buy organic meats, bake, grill or smoke and freeze into serving size portions or I have divided dishes that I will freeze a complete meal in such as meat and veggies. I even freeze pasta dishes this way such as spaghetti. Place noodles in one portion of the divided dish and the spaghetti sauce in the other portion and if you use any toppings then that will go in another divided part of the dish. Just make sure you use divided dishes with lids.

Getting prepared and organized is key to your success. Get creative and make your health a priority today.

Cristie Will

Detoxing

I detoxed for one week juicing on nothing but vegetables and a little fruit. I was so toxic that I had to get my body and mind cleansed quickly. I created and went on my "KISS 10.10.10 Diet" for a month. I would eat nothing, but RAW veggies and fruit for six months because I was still so ill. Every day got better and better.

I was so amazed at how great I felt and how my body was healing itself that I wanted more. I decided to take courses on cleansing and went on to get my certification in Intensive Cleansing to further my education to help myself and others.

I highly recommend at least a 3 day detox every three months or 1 week every six months, just to let your body rest and kick those toxins to the curb.

Detoxing is like a personal thing. So many ways to detox. I have two detox books coming out since it is one of my specialties. One is Cleansetox and it's a ten day cleanse and can be on for up to 40 days with a doctors permission. My other Detox book is on all the vast ways we can detox from food, machines, bathing, outdoors, juicing etc. We have evolved so much that I didn't realize it until all my education and experimenting with cleansing/detoxing.

Check my website for my detox classes. I run different ones at different times. www.healthtidngs.com .

7
Exercising

Activity and Exercising

The main thing with activity and exercising is just keep moving to keep your bodies system flowing and in top working order. Exercise and movement helps burn off extra calories along with getting rid of toxins through our skin via perspiration.

If you don't think you have time for exercise then at least think of ways to take extra steps such as the stairs or parking further out will bring in big benefits. When you take your 15 minute breaks at work stretch and move around benefiting your mind and body giving you that spurt of energy.

Studies show that walking can:

Reduce risk of coronary heart disease and stroke
Reduce high cholesterol
Lower blood pressure
Reduce risk of colon cancer
Reduce body fat
Help control body weight
Increase bone density and help prevent osteoporosis
Help with osteoarthritis
Reduce risk of non-insulin dependent diabetes
Help with overall flexibility
Increase mental well being
Walking Helps People Live Longer

Cristie Will

Regular participation in physical activity is associated with reduced mortality rates. (US Dept. of Health 1996). In particular, studies have shown that:

Fit and active people have approximately half the risk of cardiovascular disease compared to unfit people
Because the bones are strengthened, fit people are less likely to fall and suffer injuries such as hip fractures
Fit people are less likely to sustain injury because joints have a better range of movement and muscles are more flexible
Fit people are less prone to depression and anxiety
Fit people tend to sleep better
Fit people have better control of body weight
So in a nutshell, you can increase your chances of living longer by the simple act of walking at least 30 minutes per day.

Health Benefits of Yoga

Daily yoga practice can bring in a number of benefits to practitioners. Yoga not only helps control diseases but also plays an important role in achieving relaxation and physical fitness.

Depression and Stress: Yoga has postures for eliminating stress from the body and mind. Yogic postures such as corpse posture, child's posture, forward-bending posture, legs up the wall, cat's posture, back-bending, and headstand are considered good for eliminating depression and stress.

Yoga for a Healthy Heart: Yoga and a change in lifestyle can help in keeping a healthy heart and body. Ujjayi pranayama and bhramari pranayama are beneficial for the heart. Studies on people with coronary artery diseases have shown that including yoga along with healthy lifestyle and diet coronary artery disease was reduced drastically.

Yoga for Weight Loss: Surya Namaskara is considered to be beneficial for weight loss. Pada hasthasana and trikonasana can also be helpful in losing weight.

Health Benefits of Zumba

Zumba classes are intended to provide a large calorie burn through aerobic activity done with interval training in mind. Depending on body weight, sex, fitness level and other common physical factors, the number of calories you burn in a typical Zumba class will equal that of any fast dancing hour, like salsa, disco or jitterbug. For most people, that can add up to 400 to 600 calories burned per hour depending on age, gender and weight. Classes set up to provide intervals of intensity with music and different type of movements, class members' energy expenditure is maximized for fat-burning benefits. Fitness moves are also incorporated within Zumba dances and are great fun with high energy for the whole body.

Health Benefits of Pilates

A great thing about Pilates is it does not over-develop some parts of the body and neglect others. While Pilates training focuses on core strength, it trains the whole body. Pilate's workouts promote strength and balanced muscle development plus flexibility along with increased range of motion for the joints.

Cristie Will

Swimming

Swimming is a healthy activity that can be continued for a lifetime. The health benefits swimming offers to a swimmer are worth the effort it takes to get to the swimming pool. If you do not know how to swim, taking the time for swimming lessons or teaching yourself how to swim are well worth it. Swimming works practically all of the muscles in the body. Swimming can help develop general strength, cardiovascular fitness and endurance

Spinning

A spinning workout is an excellent way to burn some calories and relieve stress. The workout employs a stationary bike, which has various tension levels. The bike will also track your progress, so that you are motivated to continue and accomplish your fitness goals. There are numerous benefits to a spinning workout. A spinning workout of 45 minutes may allow you to burn around 500 calories.

The spinning workout may help you build some muscle tone. The workout will focus on the core muscles, as well as the buttocks and thighs. When you pedal faster, you are likely to burn fat. When you pedal slower and have a higher tension, you will work your muscles, so a mixture of both is great.

A spinning workout is a low impact exercise. This means that it won't put pressure on knees and joints, as other aerobic and running exercises can and do. Any type of exercise is known to relieve stress. However, a spinning class can be a more efficient stress reliever than most types of exercise.

Running

Like most exercises there are a number of different benefits which an individual can gain from running regularly. Some runners run simply for the joy of running but others run because there are a great deal of benefits from running. Some of these benefits include weight loss, improved cardiovascular health, improved bone health, improved mood and better coordination.

Those who are looking to lose a few pounds often find running to be one of the most effective forms of exercise for helping them to achieve their ideal body weight because it requires a great deal of energy. This great deal of energy means the body burns a larger number of calories while running. The number of calories burned while running depends on a number of factors including the individual's weight, the intensity of the workout and the gender among other factors of the runner.

Tennis

Playing tennis is great getting you moving and moving is good for the body/mind and spirit. Tennis can be played at nearly any age and skill level, because it's a low impact sport.

Stair Climbing

Whether it's an aerobic workout that feature stair climbing or just climbing the stairs they both offer a variety of benefits to your overall health. The vigorous and continuous movement of your legs and hips results in deeper breathing and increases your heartbeat, which enhances blood flow to all areas of your body. Your body releases natural pain relievers, or endorphins, during a stair climb, so you'll feel better and have less tension.

Cristie Will

Golfing

Walk a 6,500-yard course to get your heart rate up and to work up a sweat. Walking a course on a sunny day will lower harmful cholesterol and speed up your metabolism. A full round of golf can help a 200-pound man burn 350 calories or more.

Carry your own bag as you walk the course. Your golf bag may weigh 30 pounds or more. If you carry your bag, you will help create muscle mass and also make your bones stronger. Switch shoulders every other hole so you don't create too much of a strain on your neck and upper torso.

Exercise will help your body get more from sleeping than it would otherwise. Walking a course means that you are going 3 to 5 miles in a given round, which will help tire you out so you can get to sleep easier. That means you will get into a deep sleep and stay there longer than if you were not exercising. You will wake up more refreshed the next day.

8
Recipes, Tips, Guidelines and Other

Cristie's No-baking Energy Bites

Ingredients:

1 cup of dry quick Oats
2/3 cup coconut flakes
½ cup Organic Peanut butter (or your favorite nut butter)
¼ cup whole chia seeds
¼ cup whole flax seeds
1 cup Cacao Nibs
1/3 cup raw honey
1 tsp vanilla or make it other flavors

Directions:

Combine all the ingredients in large bowl. Let the mixture cool in the refrigerator for about an hour in an airtight container, then roll into 1-inch balls. These bites will not only give you energy, but will help keep you full longer.

Cristie Will

Heavenly Pecan Balls

Ingredients:

1 cup of medjool dates
1 cup of pecans
1/3 cup of Dark Chocolate (70% or higher)

Directions:

Pit the dates and place the pitted dates in food processor with the nuts and blend for about 3 minutes or until a ball forms. Divide the mixture into approximately 16 balls and freeze them about 10 minutes. Melt dark chocolate. Remove the Pecan balls from the freezer and drizzle the chocolate over the Heavenly Pecan Balls then place in the refrigerator to set then serve a little bit of Heaven.

Talk about Heaven Smoothie

Ingredients:

1/3 cup Pecans
½ lemon freshly juiced
2 medjool dates
1 cup fresh strawberries or any berries
1 cup coconut milk

Directions:

Soak the dates and nuts for about 15 Minutes. Add everything except the strawberries/berries to the blender and blend until smooth. Add strawberries until almost smooth leaving just small pieces of strawberries unblended.

Cristie Will

Healthy Special C Bar's

Ingredients:

1 cup packed medjool dates, pitted + chopped
¼ teaspoon of Celtic Sea Salt
½ cup creamy peanut butter
½ cup creamy almond butter
2-3 tablespoons of any nut butter milk
1 teaspoon maple extract (Grade B is best)
12 ounces Dark Chocolate 70% or higher
4-5 cups oats

Directions:

Grease a 9x13 inch baking dish with cooking spray or line with parchment paper. Set aside.   Add the dates and salt to the bowl of a food processor and process until they form a thick paste. Add the peanut and almond butter plus 2 tablespoons of nut milk, process until smooth and creamy. Scoop the mixture out and into a microwave safe bowl, microwaving for about 30 seconds, stir and microwave another 30 seconds or a bit longer until the mixture is warm and melted. This took me about a minute and 15 seconds. Stir in the maple extract. If the mixture is too stiff then add 1 more tablespoon of nut milk. Slowly mix oats in the peanut and almond butter mixture until thoroughly mixed. Press the mixture into the prepared baking dish in an even layer.

Microwave the chocolate on 30 to 45 second intervals, stirring every time until melted. Pour the melted chocolate over the bars in an even layer. Cover the pan and place in the fridge for 2 hours or until firm. Remove the bars 10 minutes, cut and store in the fridge. When you go to eat them or serve them they are best to leave out for 10 to 15 minutes.

Tips

Basic Setting up of your kitchen

Cutting boards are a great idea, a must and here's why. Always remember to wash with hot soapy water after each use to avoid transferring bacteria.

Wood cutting boards helps protects knife's blade.
Bamboo cutting boards helps protects knife's blade and eco-friendly.
Plastic cutting boards are durable and won't absorb moisture or odors.
Flexible cutting boards are great for light cutting. These are also great to bend, dump or push food cut up and placing where you want it to go.

Utensils

Wooden utensils will not conduct heat, need to always wash by hand and do not soak because that can cause bacteria growth.

Tongs will not conduct heat, spring action tongs stay open unless pressure applied to close them and some will lock for easier storage.

Spatulas are great with the long heat resistant handle. Be sure to choose materials that will not damage nonstick surfaces if you choose to cook with nonstick surfaces. Perforated spatulas are great to drain excess liquid or fat from foods.

Cookware

Glass and cookware with porcelain enamel coating are least reactive to foods and easiest to clean.

Cristie Will

Cast Iron is great for quick breads, pancakes, and crepes, but not recommended for soups, stews or acidic foods that require longer cooking.

Stainless steel has poor heat conductor unless layered with a highly conductible metal such as aluminum. Anodized Aluminum is toxic to the environment and not recommended. Copper is excellent conductibility though typically expensive.

Teflon can be toxic to humans, animals and the environment. If you choose to use Teflon please follow these rules for your safety. Do not use at a high temperature, do not heat dry because could cause toxic particles to become air borne, always have oil in a Teflon pan before heating, do not scratch, if you scratch discard to avoid releasing chemicals into your food and follow manufacturer's directions on cleaning to avoid damage the surface.

Steamer baskets cook vegetables quickly and water soluble vitamins stay intact. For best results look for legs ½ inch or higher, a collapsible basket so it will fit almost any size pot and folds for storage. Enamel steamers are easiest to clean. Acidic foods may leave a film on stainless steel. Can wash with brush or use dishwasher.

Bamboo Steamer cooks multiple dishes at once by stacking layers of bamboo racks. Only one burner and one pan required. Consider the lowest tier of stacked steamers cooks food faster so placed foods that require more cooking time on the bottom and place food directly on slots, or over a lettuce leaf or parchment paper.

Glass jars are ideal for storing grains, nuts, and dried legumes. Unlike plastic glass will not react with food. Glass storage containers won't stain, warp or absorb orders like plastic can. Can be used in the oven, refrigerator or freezer whereas plastic cannot be used in the oven which causes another dish to clean. Ideally buy tempered (heat treated) glass so don't have to worry about shattering if broken.

Colanders drains pasta and rinses fresh fruits and vegetables. With the holes in the colander allows air to circulate so it's great for fruits and vegetables.

Vegetable peelers peels the skin off vegetables which removes sprayed on chemicals on vegetables and or fruits.

Measuring cups measures grains, flours and liquids among other foods and are a must to have. I recommend to purchase a set with at least the four basic sizes and you can buy sets with more sizes as well.

Sharpening steel or stone to sharpen your knives. Sharp knives are safer to use than dull knives. Look for Ceramic, silicon carbide or standard steel covered with industrial diamond dust with a length of at least 6 inches long.

Pressure cooker cooks food up to three times faster than conventional cooking methods and saves energy while preserves essential vitamins and nutrients in food. Look for a highly conductive base material rich such as aluminum with spring loaded valves along with high and low settings to regulate cooking.

Santoku knives are an all-purpose kitchen chopping, slicing, and mincing of vegetables and meats. These knives are similar to a chef's knife, but lighter and smaller with straighter edge. Usuba knifes have a thin blade for cutting firm vegetables and other foods with precision and has specialized chipping such as katsuramuki (shaving a vegetable cylinder into a thin sheet).

Cristie Will

Fillet knives are flexible and used to fillet and prepare fish. Cleaver knife is large, usually rectangular heavy blade for splitting or cleaving meat and bone.

Guidelines

Simple rules for combining foods are one food per meal per group is ideal. Remember we are all different, so if you have an allergy or other reasons such has texture bothers you then substitute that food.

Proteins

Cheese	Dried Peas
Lentils	Beef
Nuts	Turkey
Dried beans	Fish
Chicken	Milk

High-Starch Foods

Grains	Yams
Potatoes	Pumpkin
Lima beans	Corn
Artichokes	Beets
Brown rice	Pasta

Greens and Low-Starch Vegetables

Endive	Cabbage
Okra	Asparagus
Peppers	Watercress
Rhubarb	Broccoli
Kohlrabi	Cucumbers
Radishes	Eggplant
Spinach	Celery
Leeks	

Avocados are best when combined with low starch veggies. Choose one kind of fruit at a time, best not to mix fruits. Only eat fruit for breakfast or in the morning. Tomatoes can be combined with low-starch veggies.

If you think you may have problems with certain foods you should keep a food diary to help narrow down problems. Keep a journal and write how certain foods make you feel.

Physical symptoms to foods examples are, headache, nausea, fatigue, insomnia, shakiness, high energy, focus, strength, bright eyes and alertness.

Emotional symptoms to foods examples are, anxious, depressed, restless, irritable, agitated energized, humorous, happy, interested and calm.

Other Eating Guidelines

Eat *before* you get hungry. Hunger is usually a sign that your blood sugar is dropping. Tendencies to overeat are more likely if you've waited too long to eat and feel overly hungry.

Eat at the right time. Eat breakfast within one to two hours of rising, lunch approximately four hours later, and dinner within six hours of lunch. If you have a day job, eat dinner before 7pm. Ironically, you should not skip meals if you are trying to lose weight. Eating properly increases your metabolism, which burns more calories.

Eat snacks. If you tend to get hungry before or between meals, have a snack. A protein snack just before bed can often help you sleep better.

Eat in peace. Distractions such as reading, watching TV, noisy environments and dinner table arguments have very harmful effects on digestion. If you are upset, calm yourself and relax before eating.

Chew well. Chewing is perhaps the most important part of the digestive process, so chew more than you think is necessary and avoid swallowing un-chewed food. Eat slowly, enjoy the flavors and textures of every bite. Stop before you're full. You'll feel full about 10 minutes after a meal if you stop eating when the food begins to lose some of its taste.

Cooking Guidelines

Use the right cooking oils. Many commonly used cooking oils are very harmful, especially when heated.

Cooking vegetables. The best way to cook vegetables is to steam them, as boiling destroys their nutrient content. Vegetables should be a little crunchy, not soggy.

Cooking meat. Ground meat should be lean and always cooked to "well done" or 160 – 165° F. Pork must be at 140 – 160° F. Other cuts can be cooked to your preference, although medium or medium rare better preserves nutrients.

Cooking poultry and fish. Remove the skin of all non-organic fowl, preferably before cooking, and use a thermometer to determine when poultry is done (165° F) or until the juice runs clear. Fish should smell a bit like the sea but fresh – it *should not* smell fishy when it is unwrapped. Make sure fish is cooked all the way through. 140° F for steaks, fillets or whole fish. When the flesh is opaque and flakes easily it is done. Shrimp should be cooked for 3 – 8 minutes depending on size. Cook them until medium rare.

Cooking Whole grains are always more healthy and nutritious than processed grains. Avoid pasta, bread, and foods made with dough. These are not whole foods but rather processed grains, and are generally not very healthy. If you do use processed grains try to purchase those that are stone ground. Grains and the oils they contain become stale and rancid over time. Avoid this by purchasing medium or small quantities from a store that refrigerates or freezes their grains. Keep your grains in the freezer. Always try to buy organic grains since non-organic are contaminated with pesticides and other chemicals.

Before cooking grains, soak them in pure water overnight then rinse them thoroughly. To cook the grain, combine it with water in a heavy pot. Do not use aluminum cookware. You may add a pinch of salt, ghee, oil or spices. Bring the grain to a boil, cover the pot, reduce heat, and simmer without stirring until the water is absorbed. Remove from heat and allow the grain to stand, still covered, for ten minutes before serving. An easy way to make whole grain cereal for breakfast is to place the grain in boiling water in a thermos the night before.

Cristie Will

Other Tidbits

I want to give you the lowdown on coffee/caffeine. Back in the day my grandparents drank coffee every day and it was good for you then. Years later coffee is supposed to be bad for you and now it's a little bit of both. Since I am a coffee drinker and absolutely love it I will start with the health benefits of coffee.

Health Benefits from Coffee/Caffeine

1. More Alert. It has been shown even low doses, 250 milligrams of caffeine, stimulates a person's alertness improving mental performance and heightening your senses.

2. Mood Elevator. As low a dose of 250 milligrams of caffeine have been reported to improve an overall sense of well-being, energy, happiness, alertness and sociability.

3. Better Concentration. Studies found that caffeine does help you perform an array of cognitive tasks, like recognizing visual patterns much faster.

4. Heightened Performance. It has been noted that caffeine allows you to exercise for longer durations without hitting exhaustion because the caffeine affects the utilization of glycogen during workouts. Glycogen is the main fuel for muscles. Once depleted, exhaustion occurs. Caffeine decreases as much as 50% of the use of glycogen during exercise thus allowing for longer workouts.

5. Less Muscle Pain. Researchers have found that caffeine potentially stimulates the release of B-endorphins and hormones that depress the sensation of pain.

6. Quicker Effects of Medications. Caffeine is known to constrict blood vessels and helps the body absorb medications more quickly, which is why it is added to some pain medications.

7. Diabetes Prevention. Coffee contains minerals and antioxidants which help prevent diabetes. Fran Hu, MD, one of the authors of The Harvard Study, theorizes it could be because caffeine stimulates muscles to burn fat and sugar more efficiently.

8. Antioxidants in caffeine help to stop free radicals from doing damage. Free radicals that are formed in a cell and not neutralized can damage the cell DNA.

9. Disease Prevention. Caffeine keeps dopamine molecules active to help prevent diseases like Parkinson's and Alzheimer's. Harvard researchers have found that men who drink four cups of caffeinated coffee a day are 50% less likely to develop Parkinson's disease and those who refrain from drinking beverages from caffeine.

10. Relief of Asthma. Drinking a moderate amount of caffeine can be therapeutic for people with asthma. Caffeine in the form of coffee could be used to prevent an asthma attack in emergencies, but it is not intended to replace medication.

Cristie Will

Possible health issues from coffee/caffeine.

1. Possible Cardiovascular Problems. About four cups of coffee or similar drink with same amount of caffeine can raise blood pressure for hours. (If you love coffee like me I would keep a log of my blood pressure readings to see if it raises my blood pressure and if it does I would give it up).

2. Stress. Drinking caffeine early in the morning can affect the body until bedtime, raising stress levels all day. Caffeine increases stress hormones and elevates a person's perception of stress. Of course to lower the stress levels it's a good idea to cut back on caffeine or completely remove caffeine from your daily intake depending on the individual.

3. Emotional Issues. By ingesting over 2 grams of caffeine daily and enters the body, the heart becomes stimulated dilating the blood vessels. Blood pressure will increase which can cause bronchial relaxation in the lungs and increased breathing.   These reactions can cause irritability, agitation, insomnia and restlessness.

4. Blood Sugar. Diabetics that are type 2 need to be award that caffeine may impair insulin's action, which causes a rise in blood sugar levels. Depending on the person, but about 2 to 2.5 cups per day may have this effect.

5. Gastrointestinal Issues. Because Caffeine is a stimulant it can increase contractions of your stomach muscles and could cause abdominal pain and diarrhea with increased bowel movements. If you have any problems or disease with your stomach/abdominal you should be extra cautious before drinking caffeine.

6. Nutritional inadequacies. Caffeine can inhibit the absorption of some nutrients and cause the urinary excretion of calcium, magnesium, potassium, iron and other minerals.

7. Male Health. Research shows that men can significantly reduce their risk for urinary and prostate problems by making dietary changes, which include eliminating coffee and caffeine.

8. Female Health. Studies show fibrocystic breast disease, osteoporosis, premenstrual syndrome, infertility problems, miscarriage, low birth weight, and menopausal problems are all heightened by caffeine. Women on birth control are at risk since they tend to have a lower ability to detoxify caffeine.

9. Aging. Caffeine tolerance may decrease with as people grow older. As we age we produce less DHEA, melatonin and other hormones. Caffeine helps to speed up this process. Caffeine will dehydrate the body, causing aging of the skin and kidneys, inhibits DNA repair, and slows the ability of the liver to detoxify foreign toxins.

10. Adrenal Exhaustion. Caffeine is stimulant that binds to adenosine receptors in the brain. Caffeine leads to a range of complex reactions that increases stimulation at the adrenal glands. This can increase a variety of health problems along the lines of inflammation and fatigue.

As you can see coffee has its good points and its bad points. Everything in life has its pros and cons too, so I encourage everyone to do their own research and to test theories on yourself, only if not harmful though, to see works for you. We are all different and what works for you may not work for someone else even in the same family. It will be up to the individual and your health care professional if drinking coffee is ok for you.

Cristie Will

With this fast paced world things change and what use to be ok to consume could change and not be ok to consume later. A great example of this is wheat. The wheat our ancestors ate is not the same as the wheat today and this is why people are having more and more health issues with wheat. If you go out and do your research on wheat you will find the DNA structure of wheat has been changed dozens and dozens of times making the DNA totally different. The DNA of wheat has been changed so much to give it better taste and consistency. This process has taken years and is probably ongoing as other products are as well.

The eight causes of Cravings

1. Lack of Primary Foods such as being in a dissatisfied relationship, being bored or being stressed just to name a few reasons. This can cause emotional eating causing a temporary substitute for this dissatisfaction or yearning.

2. Lack of water will send the message you are hungry if you are dehydrated.

3. Yin-Yang imbalance is simply food imbalances like eating a diet too rich in sugar.

4. Inside/Out. Cravings often times can come from foods that we recently ate or foods from childhood or our ancestors. The best way to fix this is to eat a healthier version of what we at in our childhoods or from our ancestors.

5. Seasonal. The body craves foods to help balance the elements of the season. In the spring we crave detoxifying foods likes salads or citrus and in the fall like squash, onions and nuts. The cravings are different for summer and winter.

6. Lack of Nutrients. If your body has inadequate nutrients it will cause cravings. An example would be inadequate mineral levels produce salt cravings.

7. Hormonal. Fluctuating hormone levels will cause cravings as well.

8. Self-Sabotage. When things are going really well, sometimes we self-sabotage. We then crave foods creating more cravings to balance ourselves. This often happens from low blood sugar and can result in strong mood swings.

9

Steps I took for my Transformation

Starting a journey to lose 200 pounds is quite scary and I knew I needed some momentum. In light of needing a quick easy weight loss I came up with my KISS 10.10.10 Diet Plan. This started my journey and I still use this with a little tweaking as you will see. This will help jumpstart your journey to lose weight once and for all.

1.   Commit and keep track with a journal (My journal "KISS 10.10.10. Diet").
2.   Drink 64 ounces of water a day.
3.   Eat 50% of veggies and fruit as your daily food intake.
4.   Stick to consuming 1,000 calories a day.
5.   Walk 20 minutes 5 days a week.
6.   Cut out processed foods. (If it comes in a package of any kind don't eat it)
7.   Meditate 15 minutes every night visualizing yourself thin.
8.   Plan your meals for 10 days, prepare ahead to ensure success.
9.   Take a vitamin supplement and a probiotic in capsule form.
10. Take 10 deep breaths 3 times a day to aid in weight loss.

Cristie's steps to Vibrant and Healthy Weight Loss today

- Commit is first step I was literally so sick and tired of living, looking and being unhealthy.
- I quit smoking. Gave myself time to get through all the road blocks of ditching smoking.
- I cleaned out pantry, freezer and refrigerator of toxic food.
- Started juicing to cleanse my body of toxic waste
- Started Meditating and Deep Breathing. First once a day then added morning and night.
- Added Supplements
- Started Visualization seeing myself thin to win. I would visualize in the morning upon waking up and in the evening when going to bed. See Chapter 5 for visualization guided meditations to use or use your own.
- Added spoken daily affirmations (remember what we speak about seems to show up in our life). I have found that spoken affirmations are much more effective than writing them out. (If you want and have time then you can write them too).
- Exercising – Walking only at first. I built up to about 4 miles three days a week. After six months into my other steps listed above I added Walking. It was so difficult to move around I decided I would give myself six months before exercising. After losing about 150 pounds I started yoga, golf, running and other activities I dabbled in.
- Wanted to have a new career in doing what I love, so I changed careers.
- I went back to school and enrolled in The Instituted of Integrative Nutrition. My education helped me find and realize my missing dots.
- Evaluate and change my toxic relationships
- My Spirituality was missing, so I turned to my Creator for help and Guidance.

I now know why diets fail and what it takes to lose the weight and be healthy. Balance in our lives is necessary or it will always be a struggle. To have balance you need healthy food, relationships, career, exercise and spirituality. With us all being different our dots will be different, but it's the same main things in life that we need.

For me and my experience it takes all these steps, (smoking and menopause don't count if not going through menopause or smoke). The best way is to incorporate a couple of these things at a time and when the time is right start adding more changes.

Anything worthwhile takes time. I can help you with this and together we can reach your goals.

I strive to be 100% healthy and eating all the right things, but I am human and don't always. I live the 80/20 rule, 80% perfect healthy eating and 20% allowance. I plan to be 90/10 by June 1, 2015. I will stay at the 90/10 because my view is you have to live and if you can live 90/10 then you can detox the 10% away.

Cristie's Daily Routine

First thing is I meditate, visualize and pray each morning.

Morning:

2 cups of coffee with creamer/honey.
I don't get the nonfat or anything like that. Sometimes as a treat I will buy the creamer that is not the healthiest. This is in my 80/20 and soon to be in my 90/10. Different articles saying coffee isn't bad and some it's good. I figure in moderation and its ok or at least for me.

Smoothie in my Vitamix.
I prefer smoothies over juicing because I believe we are leaving too much good nutrition behind in the pulp. With the Vitamix or a really good blender you blend it all, except for some nuts and seeds like the apple seeds are bad so I cut those out. (See Recipes under Dot 8, Gorgeous Green Smoothie).

Veggie Egg Omelet one or two days a week instead of the smoothie.
I mix 2 eggs (the whole egg, organic) in with veggies and spices, (the veggies will vary according to what I have. Spices will vary too. Like if I am making a Mexican omelet I will add Mexican spices like Cumin and Chili power. I will have these recipes in my cookbook coming up. 2 slices of Great Harvest Bread when I want to make it a sandwich.

Slice up apple with peanut butter or some kind of nut butter with my Omelet. I will add dried fruit as well like blueberries, cherries or cranberries. Sometimes I will slice a banana vertically and add nut butter to the banana and sprinkle some dried fruit this way just like my apples.

Cristie Will

Last but not least I just have a medium sized fruit bowl for the morning. Change it up so it doesn't get boring and the same old thing. Take my supplements with my breakfast.

Exercise for 30 minutes to an hour.

Lunch

Bowl of Soup or cup of soup and a Salad.
If I have a cup of soup then I add a large salad and if I have a bowl of soup then I add a small salad. My soups will vary. I make homemade soup. It can range from Vegetable to Bean soup. I try and stay away from pasta in my soups, but I will add a little brown, black rice or wild rice is best. I occasionally will have chicken and wild rice soup. I am not totally plant based, but close. I like to eat meat like a condiment, very little or maybe once a week some chicken or fish. I eat a little pork or beef about once every two months.

My salads will consist of lots of things from, all the green salad, tomatoes, celery, cucumbers, bell peppers, hot peppers, carrots, rice, beans, lentils, dried fruits, fresh fruits, all kinds of nuts and seeds. I always use some kind of Balsamic Vinegar and either olive oil, avocado oil or coconut oil. I do use spices along with a little sea salt and pepper.

Take rest of my supplements

Dinner

Large Salad and Veggie Plate.
Just as my lunch my salad will have an array of things, but it will be a large one and if I feel like I want more then I will bake some veggies with spices and nutritional yeast….yummy. I sometimes will bake veggies

with a little oil and spices in the oven and absolutely delicious. I drink water most of the time, but sometimes will have tea with honey.

Living in the 80/20 rule I allow myself to have Pizza once a month or I go have full blown Mexican food. When I have pizza I get the thin crust and gluten free when I can. I will get vegetarian or limit my meat to one kind. When I eat Mexican food I will limit my bread choices. I will get a Taco Salad with beans no meat or I may have a burrito with tortilla or sometimes I have burrito in a bowl.

Bedtime

Read for about an hour and journal. Just before bed I meditate, visualize and pray each night.

I started out eating 1,000 calories a day, but now as a rule I do not count calories because it's no longer necessary with my new healthy habits and way of life. I do watch my intake though. It's easier than it used to be. I eat healthy for the most part now and don't have near the cravings.

I make sure my meat is organic, (no hormones, antibiotics, non GMO, grass fed and grass finished). Same thing with my bread. I eat Great Harvest Bread because they use honey and everything is natural. There is typically only 5 ingredients in their sandwich bread or I buy gluten free at Great Harvest as well.

10
30 Days Journal & Diet
Tracker

PERSONAL GOALS

Start Date: _____   End Date: _____

My Goals: _____

_____

_____

My Plans: _____

_____

_____

Daily Food Targets

| calories | fat | carbs | fiber |
| protein | | | |

My Statistics

GOAL	RECORD ONE OR MORE	BEFORE	AFTER	NET +/-
	weight			
	cholesterol level			
	blood pressure			
	MEASUREMENTS:			
	chest			
	waist			
	hip			
	neck			
	upper arms			
	thighs			
	calves			

Before Pictures Here

After Pictures Here

DAY #:_____

Meal 1	Portion Sizes	Fat	Calories	Carbs	Protein
TOTALS					
Satisfied after eating?					

Meal 2	Portion Sizes	Fat	Calories	Carbs	Protein
TOTALS					
Satisfied after eating?					

Notes

Meal 3	Portion Sizes	Fat	Calories	Carbs	Protein
TOTALS					
Satisfied after eating?					

Meal 4	Portion Sizes	Fat	Calories	Carbs	Protein
TOTALS					
Satisfied after eating?					

Meal 5	Portion Sizes	Fat	Calories	Carbs	Protein
TOTALS					
Satisfied after eating?					

DAY #:_____

Meal 1	Portion Sizes	Fat	Calories	Carbs	Protein
TOTALS					
Satisfied after eating?					
Meal 2	Portion Sizes	Fat	Calories	Carbs	Protein
TOTALS					
Satisfied after eating?					

Notes

Meal 3	Portion Sizes	Fat	Calories	Carbs	Protein
TOTALS					
Satisfied after eating?					

Meal 4	Portion Sizes	Fat	Calories	Carbs	Protein
TOTALS					
Satisfied after eating?					

Meal 5	Portion Sizes	Fat	Calories	Carbs	Protein
TOTALS					
Satisfied after eating?					

DAY #:_____

Meal 1	Portion Sizes	Fat	Calories	Carbs	Protein
TOTALS					
Satisfied after eating?					

Meal 2	Portion Sizes	Fat	Calories	Carbs	Protein
TOTALS					
Satisfied after eating?					

Notes

Meal 3	Portion Sizes	Fat	Calories	Carbs	Protein
TOTALS					
Satisfied after eating?					

Meal 4	Portion Sizes	Fat	Calories	Carbs	Protein
TOTALS					
Satisfied after eating?					

Meal 5	Portion Sizes	Fat	Calories	Carbs	Protein
TOTALS					
Satisfied after eating?					

DAY #:_____

Meal 1	Portion Sizes	Fat	Calories	Carbs	Protein
TOTALS					
Satisfied after eating?					

Meal 2	Portion Sizes	Fat	Calories	Carbs	Protein
TOTALS					
Satisfied after eating?					

Notes

Meal 3	Portion Sizes	Fat	Calories	Carbs	Protein
TOTALS					
Satisfied after eating?					

Meal 4	Portion Sizes	Fat	Calories	Carbs	Protein
TOTALS					
Satisfied after eating?					

Meal 5	Portion Sizes	Fat	Calories	Carbs	Protein
TOTALS					
Satisfied after eating?					

DAY #:_____

Meal 1	Portion Sizes	Fat	Calories	Carbs	Protein
TOTALS					
Satisfied after eating?					

Meal 2	Portion Sizes	Fat	Calories	Carbs	Protein
TOTALS					
Satisfied after eating?					

Notes

Meal 3	Portion Sizes	Fat	Calories	Carbs	Protein
TOTALS					
Satisfied after eating?					

Meal 4	Portion Sizes	Fat	Calories	Carbs	Protein
TOTALS					
Satisfied after eating?					

Meal 5	Portion Sizes	Fat	Calories	Carbs	Protein
TOTALS					
Satisfied after eating?					

DAY #:_____

Meal 1	Portion Sizes	Fat	Calories	Carbs	Protein
TOTALS					
Satisfied after eating?					

Meal 2	Portion Sizes	Fat	Calories	Carbs	Protein
TOTALS					
Satisfied after eating?					

Notes

Meal 3	Portion Sizes	Fat	Calories	Carbs	Protein
TOTALS					
Satisfied after eating?					

Meal 4	Portion Sizes	Fat	Calories	Carbs	Protein
TOTALS					
Satisfied after eating?					

Meal 5	Portion Sizes	Fat	Calories	Carbs	Protein
TOTALS					
Satisfied after eating?					

DAY #:_____

Meal 1	Portion Sizes	Fat	Calories	Carbs	Protein
TOTALS					
Satisfied after eating?					

Meal 2	Portion Sizes	Fat	Calories	Carbs	Protein
TOTALS					
Satisfied after eating?					

Notes

Meal 3	Portion Sizes	Fat	Calories	Carbs	Protein
TOTALS					
Satisfied after eating?					

Meal 4	Portion Sizes	Fat	Calories	Carbs	Protein
TOTALS					
Satisfied after eating?					

Meal 5	Portion Sizes	Fat	Calories	Carbs	Protein
TOTALS					
Satisfied after eating?					

DAY #:_____

Meal 1	Portion Sizes	Fat	Calories	Carbs	Protein
TOTALS					
Satisfied after eating?					
Meal 2	Portion Sizes	Fat	Calories	Carbs	Protein
TOTALS					
Satisfied after eating?					

Notes

Meal 3	Portion Sizes	Fat	Calories	Carbs	Protein
TOTALS					
Satisfied after eating?					

Meal 4	Portion Sizes	Fat	Calories	Carbs	Protein
TOTALS					
Satisfied after eating?					

Meal 5	Portion Sizes	Fat	Calories	Carbs	Protein
TOTALS					
Satisfied after eating?					

DAY #: _____

Meal 1	Portion Sizes	Fat	Calories	Carbs	Protein
TOTALS					
Satisfied after eating?					

Meal 2	Portion Sizes	Fat	Calories	Carbs	Protein
TOTALS					
Satisfied after eating?					

Notes

Meal 3	Portion Sizes	Fat	Calories	Carbs	Protein
TOTALS					
Satisfied after eating?					

Meal 4	Portion Sizes	Fat	Calories	Carbs	Protein
TOTALS					
Satisfied after eating?					

Meal 5	Portion Sizes	Fat	Calories	Carbs	Protein
TOTALS					
Satisfied after eating?					

DAY #:_____

Meal 1	Portion Sizes	Fat	Calories	Carbs	Protein
TOTALS					
Satisfied after eating?					

Meal 2	Portion Sizes	Fat	Calories	Carbs	Protein
TOTALS					
Satisfied after eating?					

Notes

Meal 3	Portion Sizes	Fat	Calories	Carbs	Protein
TOTALS					
Satisfied after eating?					

Meal 4	Portion Sizes	Fat	Calories	Carbs	Protein
TOTALS					
Satisfied after eating?					

Meal 5	Portion Sizes	Fat	Calories	Carbs	Protein
TOTALS					
Satisfied after eating?					

DAY #:_____

Meal 1	Portion Sizes	Fat	Calories	Carbs	Protein
TOTALS					
Satisfied after eating?					

Meal 2	Portion Sizes	Fat	Calories	Carbs	Protein
TOTALS					
Satisfied after eating?					

Notes

Meal 3	Portion Sizes	Fat	Calories	Carbs	Protein
TOTALS					
Satisfied after eating?					

Meal 4	Portion Sizes	Fat	Calories	Carbs	Protein
TOTALS					
Satisfied after eating?					

Meal 5	Portion Sizes	Fat	Calories	Carbs	Protein
TOTALS					
Satisfied after eating?					

DAY #:_____

Meal 1	Portion Sizes	Fat	Calories	Carbs	Protein
TOTALS					
Satisfied after eating?					
Meal 2	Portion Sizes	Fat	Calories	Carbs	Protein
TOTALS					
Satisfied after eating?					

Notes

Meal 3	Portion Sizes	Fat	Calories	Carbs	Protein
TOTALS					

Satisfied after eating?

Meal 4	Portion Sizes	Fat	Calories	Carbs	Protein
TOTALS					

Satisfied after eating?

Meal 5	Portion Sizes	Fat	Calories	Carbs	Protein
TOTALS					

Satisfied after eating?

DAY #:_____

Meal 1	Portion Sizes	Fat	Calories	Carbs	Protein
TOTALS					
Satisfied after eating?					

Meal 2	Portion Sizes	Fat	Calories	Carbs	Protein
TOTALS					
Satisfied after eating?					

Notes

Meal 3	Portion Sizes	Fat	Calories	Carbs	Protein
TOTALS					
Satisfied after eating?					

Meal 4	Portion Sizes	Fat	Calories	Carbs	Protein
TOTALS					
Satisfied after eating?					

Meal 5	Portion Sizes	Fat	Calories	Carbs	Protein
TOTALS					
Satisfied after eating?					

DAY #:_____

Meal 1	Portion Sizes	Fat	Calories	Carbs	Protein
TOTALS					
Satisfied after eating?					

Meal 2	Portion Sizes	Fat	Calories	Carbs	Protein
TOTALS					
Satisfied after eating?					

Notes

Meal 3	Portion Sizes	Fat	Calories	Carbs	Protein
TOTALS					

Satisfied after eating?	

Meal 4	Portion Sizes	Fat	Calories	Carbs	Protein
TOTALS					

Satisfied after eating?	

Meal 5	Portion Sizes	Fat	Calories	Carbs	Protein
TOTALS					

Satisfied after eating?	

DAY #:_____

Meal 1	Portion Sizes	Fat	Calories	Carbs	Protein
TOTALS					
Satisfied after eating?					

Meal 2	Portion Sizes	Fat	Calories	Carbs	Protein
TOTALS					
Satisfied after eating?					

Notes

Meal 3	Portion Sizes	Fat	Calories	Carbs	Protein
TOTALS					
Satisfied after eating?					

Meal 4	Portion Sizes	Fat	Calories	Carbs	Protein
TOTALS					
Satisfied after eating?					

Meal 5	Portion Sizes	Fat	Calories	Carbs	Protein
TOTALS					
Satisfied after eating?					

DAY #:_____

Meal 1	Portion Sizes	Fat	Calories	Carbs	Protein
TOTALS					
Satisfied after eating?					

Meal 2	Portion Sizes	Fat	Calories	Carbs	Protein
TOTALS					
Satisfied after eating?					

Notes

Meal 3	Portion Sizes	Fat	Calories	Carbs	Protein
TOTALS					
Satisfied after eating?					

Meal 4	Portion Sizes	Fat	Calories	Carbs	Protein
TOTALS					
Satisfied after eating?					

Meal 5	Portion Sizes	Fat	Calories	Carbs	Protein
TOTALS					
Satisfied after eating?					

DAY #:_____

Meal 1	Portion Sizes	Fat	Calories	Carbs	Protein
TOTALS					
Satisfied after eating?					

Meal 2	Portion Sizes	Fat	Calories	Carbs	Protein
TOTALS					
Satisfied after eating?					

Notes

Meal 3	Portion Sizes	Fat	Calories	Carbs	Protein
TOTALS					
Satisfied after eating?					

Meal 4	Portion Sizes	Fat	Calories	Carbs	Protein
TOTALS					
Satisfied after eating?					

Meal 5	Portion Sizes	Fat	Calories	Carbs	Protein
TOTALS					
Satisfied after eating?					

DAY #:_____

Meal 1	Portion Sizes	Fat	Calories	Carbs	Protein
TOTALS					
Satisfied after eating?					

Meal 2	Portion Sizes	Fat	Calories	Carbs	Protein
TOTALS					
Satisfied after eating?					

Notes

Meal 3	Portion Sizes	Fat	Calories	Carbs	Protein
TOTALS					
Satisfied after eating?					

Meal 4	Portion Sizes	Fat	Calories	Carbs	Protein
TOTALS					
Satisfied after eating?					

Meal 5	Portion Sizes	Fat	Calories	Carbs	Protein
TOTALS					
Satisfied after eating?					

DAY #:_____

Meal 1	Portion Sizes	Fat	Calories	Carbs	Protein
TOTALS					
Satisfied after eating?					
Meal 2	Portion Sizes	Fat	Calories	Carbs	Protein
TOTALS					
Satisfied after eating?					

Notes

Meal 3	Portion Sizes	Fat	Calories	Carbs	Protein
TOTALS					
Satisfied after eating?					

Meal 4	Portion Sizes	Fat	Calories	Carbs	Protein
TOTALS					
Satisfied after eating?					

Meal 5	Portion Sizes	Fat	Calories	Carbs	Protein
TOTALS					
Satisfied after eating?					

DAY #:_____

Meal 1	Portion Sizes	Fat	Calories	Carbs	Protein
TOTALS					
Satisfied after eating?					

Meal 2	Portion Sizes	Fat	Calories	Carbs	Protein
TOTALS					
Satisfied after eating?					

Notes

Meal 3	Portion Sizes	Fat	Calories	Carbs	Protein
TOTALS					

Satisfied after eating?

Meal 4	Portion Sizes	Fat	Calories	Carbs	Protein
TOTALS					

Satisfied after eating?

Meal 5	Portion Sizes	Fat	Calories	Carbs	Protein
TOTALS					

Satisfied after eating?

DAY #:_____

Meal 1	Portion Sizes	Fat	Calories	Carbs	Protein
TOTALS					
Satisfied after eating?					

Meal 2	Portion Sizes	Fat	Calories	Carbs	Protein
TOTALS					
Satisfied after eating?					

Notes

Meal 3	Portion Sizes	Fat	Calories	Carbs	Protein
TOTALS					
Satisfied after eating?					

Meal 4	Portion Sizes	Fat	Calories	Carbs	Protein
TOTALS					
Satisfied after eating?					

Meal 5	Portion Sizes	Fat	Calories	Carbs	Protein
TOTALS					
Satisfied after eating?					

DAY #:_____

Meal 1	Portion Sizes	Fat	Calories	Carbs	Protein
TOTALS					
Satisfied after eating?					
Meal 2	Portion Sizes	Fat	Calories	Carbs	Protein
TOTALS					
Satisfied after eating?					

Notes

Meal 3	Portion Sizes	Fat	Calories	Carbs	Protein
TOTALS					
Satisfied after eating?					

Meal 4	Portion Sizes	Fat	Calories	Carbs	Protein
TOTALS					
Satisfied after eating?					

Meal 5	Portion Sizes	Fat	Calories	Carbs	Protein
TOTALS					
Satisfied after eating?					

DAY #:_____

Meal 1	Portion Sizes	Fat	Calories	Carbs	Protein
TOTALS					
Satisfied after eating?					

Meal 2	Portion Sizes	Fat	Calories	Carbs	Protein
TOTALS					
Satisfied after eating?					

Notes

Meal 3	Portion Sizes	Fat	Calories	Carbs	Protein
TOTALS					
Satisfied after eating?					

Meal 4	Portion Sizes	Fat	Calories	Carbs	Protein
TOTALS					
Satisfied after eating?					

Meal 5	Portion Sizes	Fat	Calories	Carbs	Protein
TOTALS					
Satisfied after eating?					

DAY #:_____

Meal 1	Portion Sizes	Fat	Calories	Carbs	Protein
TOTALS					
Satisfied after eating?					

Meal 2	Portion Sizes	Fat	Calories	Carbs	Protein
TOTALS					
Satisfied after eating?					

Notes

Meal 3	Portion Sizes	Fat	Calories	Carbs	Protein
TOTALS					
Satisfied after eating?					

Meal 4	Portion Sizes	Fat	Calories	Carbs	Protein
TOTALS					
Satisfied after eating?					

Meal 5	Portion Sizes	Fat	Calories	Carbs	Protein
TOTALS					
Satisfied after eating?					

DAY #:_____

Meal 1	Portion Sizes	Fat	Calories	Carbs	Protein
TOTALS					
Satisfied after eating?					

Meal 2	Portion Sizes	Fat	Calories	Carbs	Protein
TOTALS					
Satisfied after eating?					

Notes

Meal 3	Portion Sizes	Fat	Calories	Carbs	Protein
TOTALS					
Satisfied after eating?					

Meal 4	Portion Sizes	Fat	Calories	Carbs	Protein
TOTALS					
Satisfied after eating?					

Meal 5	Portion Sizes	Fat	Calories	Carbs	Protein
TOTALS					
Satisfied after eating?					

DAY #:_____

Meal 1	Portion Sizes	Fat	Calories	Carbs	Protein
TOTALS					
Satisfied after eating?					

Meal 2	Portion Sizes	Fat	Calories	Carbs	Protein
TOTALS					
Satisfied after eating?					

Notes

Meal 3	Portion Sizes	Fat	Calories	Carbs	Protein
TOTALS					
Satisfied after eating?					

Meal 4	Portion Sizes	Fat	Calories	Carbs	Protein
TOTALS					
Satisfied after eating?					

Meal 5	Portion Sizes	Fat	Calories	Carbs	Protein
TOTALS					
Satisfied after eating?					

DAY #:_____

Meal 1	Portion Sizes	Fat	Calories	Carbs	Protein
TOTALS					
Satisfied after eating?					
Meal 2	Portion Sizes	Fat	Calories	Carbs	Protein
TOTALS					
Satisfied after eating?					

Notes

Meal 3	Portion Sizes	Fat	Calories	Carbs	Protein
TOTALS					
Satisfied after eating?					

Meal 4	Portion Sizes	Fat	Calories	Carbs	Protein
TOTALS					
Satisfied after eating?					

Meal 5	Portion Sizes	Fat	Calories	Carbs	Protein
TOTALS					
Satisfied after eating?					

DAY #:_____

Meal 1	Portion Sizes	Fat	Calories	Carbs	Protein
TOTALS					
Satisfied after eating?					

Meal 2	Portion Sizes	Fat	Calories	Carbs	Protein
TOTALS					
Satisfied after eating?					

Notes

Meal 3	Portion Sizes	Fat	Calories	Carbs	Protein
TOTALS					
Satisfied after eating?					

Meal 4	Portion Sizes	Fat	Calories	Carbs	Protein
TOTALS					
Satisfied after eating?					

Meal 5	Portion Sizes	Fat	Calories	Carbs	Protein
TOTALS					
Satisfied after eating?					

DAY #:_____

Meal 1	Portion Sizes	Fat	Calories	Carbs	Protein
TOTALS					
Satisfied after eating?					

Meal 2	Portion Sizes	Fat	Calories	Carbs	Protein
TOTALS					
Satisfied after eating?					

Notes

Meal 3	Portion Sizes	Fat	Calories	Carbs	Protein
TOTALS					
Satisfied after eating?					

Meal 4	Portion Sizes	Fat	Calories	Carbs	Protein
TOTALS					
Satisfied after eating?					

Meal 5	Portion Sizes	Fat	Calories	Carbs	Protein
TOTALS					
Satisfied after eating?					

DAY #:_____

Meal 1	Portion Sizes	Fat	Calories	Carbs	Protein
TOTALS					
Satisfied after eating?					

Meal 2	Portion Sizes	Fat	Calories	Carbs	Protein
TOTALS					
Satisfied after eating?					

Notes

Meal 3	Portion Sizes	Fat	Calories	Carbs	Protein
TOTALS					
Satisfied after eating?					

Meal 4	Portion Sizes	Fat	Calories	Carbs	Protein
TOTALS					
Satisfied after eating?					

Meal 5	Portion Sizes	Fat	Calories	Carbs	Protein
TOTALS					
Satisfied after eating?					

11
Suggested Reading and Links

http://www.healthtidings.com/

http://www.cbwill.com/

http://www.integrativenutrition.com/

www.thedanielplan.com

http://drhyman.com/

http://www.doctoryourself.com/

http://www.foodmatters.tv/

http://www.doctoroz.com/

http://www.mercola.com/

Conclusion

Simply put, no two fingerprints are alike, so no two people are alike. This is why no diets work the same on anyone. We are bio individuals making our minds, bodies and spirits unique.

This is the only science that has the research that states an answer and another research on the same thing giving a completely different answer and the reason being is what works for one person may not work for the next.

Also, this is why science/research can show why being a Vegan is the best and science/research can come back with points that eating meat is healthier. All points on both sides are true. The reason for the truth is because it's best for some to be Vegan and some to be Meat Eaters such as the Primal or Paleo way.

Some researchers conclude dairy is bad and it's true, but for only some people. Same thing with wheat, but again for only some people.

At the end of the day, with my education, research and testing on myself I have found what works for me and that none of the so called magic pills/powders works. None of the diets work long term without adjustments for me and each of us.

Our creator gave us amazing bodies that knows how to heal itself, when to sleep, when to wake up and when to use the restroom at the same time maintaining a 98.6 degrees. Your heart never missing a beat while lungs always breathing and knows the miracles of having a child. Our creator gave us foods to choose from for our bodies and that's why food can heal if given the right foods. Give your body, mind and spirt what is needed and the gifts you will receive from doing this will far outweigh anything you ever dreamed possible. It will cause a domino effect with

Conclusion Continued

one great thing after another starting to happen and change for you. First off your health will start to get better, you will look great, then your self-esteem goes way up, you now have confidence to take chances and as you take those chances doors open up for things and opportunities to come your way.

Another gift you will receive from giving yourself what is needed and that is you will be an example and others will follow. This is how you become a part of the domino effect.

Thank you for buying this book and reading it. I hope you take the time for yourself and make the necessary changes you so deeply desire, need and deserve. You can be and have anything you want if you just take that first step to change and follow through. I not only lost the weight, quit smoking, went through menopause, lost my husband to cancer and made a complete career change in my 50's and you can too.

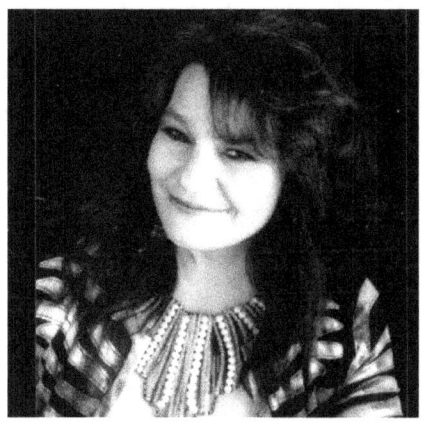

Cristie Will, CHC, CIC
Author

Cristie Will – An Accountant who traded in her calculator to master her calling to help people lose weight the healthy way and to gain optimal health and wellness. She decided to do this after losing her husband to lung cancer in 2012. Due to her own life threatening health issues she turned her health around losing 200 pounds and ditching all medications.

Cristie lives in Johnstown, Colorado and has helped others reach optimal health and wellness. She has written and published 5 Cookbooks. She has two grown children Lauren and Josh and four grandchildren.

Cristie received her training as a Certified Health Coach from the Institute for Integrative Nutrition training and training for her Cleansing Intensive Certification as a Cleansing Detoxing Coach from the Wild Rose College under Dr. Terry Willard CIH, PHD.

Cristie Will

Reviews

I highly recommend this book Fat GONE! After reading this book, not only did it inspire me to access my own health, but her story is so heartwarming. She has been there and done it throughout her life with weight issues. This book is chalked full of information from a few Recipes, steps on how she did it along with invaluable information that I will use time and time again instead of running to the computer to look up. The Tracker Journal is a great tool too.

Belinda Shelton

Finally a book that ties in everything from food, exercise, relationships, careers, spirituality along with steps to take to take control of your health. This book is an invaluable tool. It has just the right amount of information at a time to implement.

Deann Skinner

Citations/Index/Resources

Sources:

Centers for Disease Control and Prevention. Smoking-Attributable Mortality, Years of Potential Life Lost, and Productivity Losses — United States, 2000–2004. Morbidity and Mortality Weekly Report. November 14, 2008; 57(45):1226–28.

1.   Centers for Disease Control and Prevention. National Center for Chronic Disease Prevention and Health Promotion. Tobacco Information and Prevention Source (TIPS). Tobacco Use in the United States. January 27, 2004.

2.   Centers for Disease Control and Prevention. National Center for Health Statistics. National Health Interview Survey Raw Data, 2009. Analysis by the American Lung Association, Research and Program Services Division using SPSS and SUDAAN software.

3.   Centers for Disease Control and Prevention. Cigarette Smoking Attributable Morbidity—United States, 2000. Morbidity and Mortality Weekly Report. September 5, 2003; 52(35).

4.   U.S Department of Health and Human Services. Health Consequences of Smoking: A Report of the Surgeon General, 2004.

5.   Centers for Disease Control and Prevention. National Center for Health Statistics. National Health Interview Survey Raw Data, 2009. Analysis by the American Lung Association, Research and Program Services Division using SPSS and SUDAAN software.

6.   Ibid.

7.   Ibid.

8.   Centers for Disease Control and Prevention. Youth Risk Behavior Surveillance — United States, 2009. Morbidity and Mortality Weekly Report. June 4, 2010; 59(SS-05).

9.   Centers for Disease Control and Prevention. Office on Smoking and Health. National Youth Tobacco Survey, 2009. Analysis by the American Lung Association, Research and Program Services Division using SPSS software.

10.   U.S Department of Health and Human Services. Women and Smoking: A Report of the Surgeon General, 2001.

11.   Centers for Disease Control and Prevention. National Center for Health Statistics. National Vital Statistics Reports. Births: Final Data for 2005. December 5, 2007; (56)5.

12.   Centers for Disease Control and Prevention. State Estimates of Neonatal Health-Care Costs Associated with Maternal Smoking—United States, 1996. Morbidity and Mortality Weekly Report. October 8, 2004; 53(39).

13.   National Institute of Drug Abuse. Research Report on Nicotine: Addiction, August 2001.

14.   Centers for Disease Control and Prevention. National Center for Health Statistics. National Health Interview Survey Raw Data, 2009. Analysis by the American Lung Association, Research and Program Services Division using SPSS and SUDAAN software.

15.   Centers for Disease Control and Prevention. Smoking and Tobacco Use. You Can Quit Smoking. Accessed on October 2, 2007.

16.   Fiore MC, Jaen CR, Baker TB, et al. Treating Tobacco Use and Dependence: 2008 Update. Clinical Practice Guideline. Rockville, MD: U.S. Department of Health and Human Services. Public Health Service. May 2008.

17.   Ibid.

18.   U.S Department of Health and Human Services. How Tobacco Smoke Causes Disease: The Biology and Behavioral Basis for Smoking-Attributable Disease: A Report of the Surgeon General, 2010.

Note: Racial and ethnic minority terminology reflects those terms used by the Centers for Disease Control and Prevention.

Source for Menopause: Information obtained from the Mayo Clinic. http://www.mayoclinic.org/diseases-conditions/menopause/basics/symptoms/con-20019726

Source for information is from my education at IIN and hard knocks.

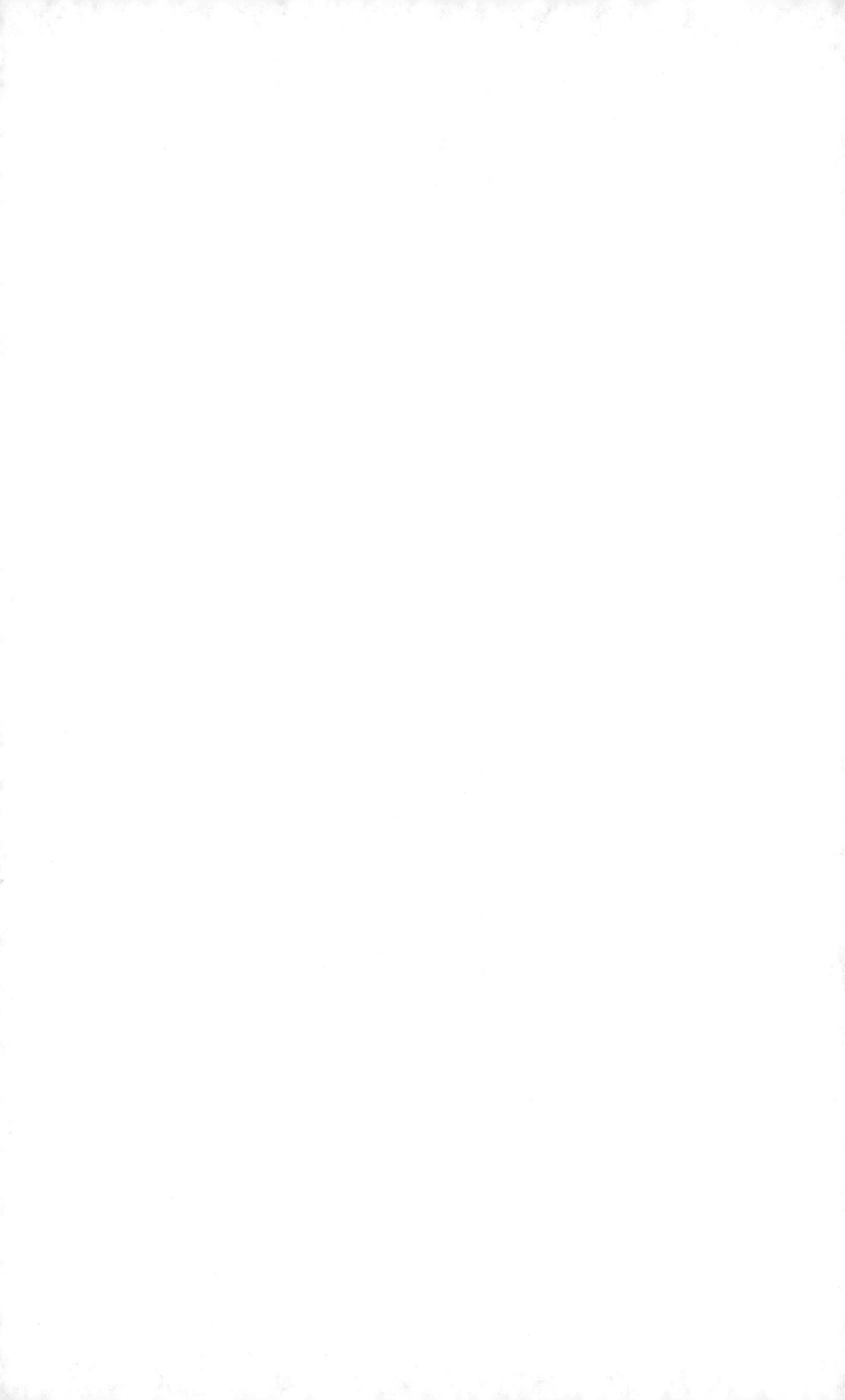